THE POSTURALITY OF THE PERSON

A Guide to Postural Education and Therapy

Ron Dennis, Ed.D.

Posturality Press
Atlanta

THE POSTURALITY OF THE PERSON
A Guide to Postural Education and Therapy

Copyright © 2013 by Ronald J. Dennis

ISBN 978-0-9882525-0-9

Published by
   Alexander Technique of Atlanta/Posturality Press
   Ronald J. Dennis, Proprietor
   Websites: www.posturality.com
             www.posturecounts.com
   Email: rondennis@compuserve.com

The content of this book is not to be construed as a substitute for medical examination, diagnosis, and treatment. Any person with symptoms seemingly related to the materials presented herein is well-advised to consult with a physician. The author-publisher disclaims any liability for the use of this book in any way other than for information and education.

"... a Book is a Person not a Thing"
W. N. P. Barbellion
The Journal of a Disappointed Man

Before you embark on any path ask the question: Does this path have a heart? ... A path without a heart is never enjoyable. You have to work hard even to take it. On the other hand, a path with heart is easy; it does not make you work at liking it. ... For me there is only the traveling on the paths that have a heart, on any path that may have a heart. There I travel, and the only worthwhile challenge for me is to traverse its full length.

From *The Teachings of Don Juan*
A Yaqui Way of Knowledge
by Carlos Castaneda

If you lose the spirit of repetition, your practice will become quite difficult.

Shunryu Suzuki
Zen Mind, Beginner's Mind

In letters of gold on T'ang's bathtub:
AS THE SUN MAKES IT NEW
DAY BY DAY MAKE IT NEW
YET AGAIN MAKE IT NEW

From *Confucius: The Great Digest*
by Ezra Pound

To Judith Leibowitz (1920–1990)
my principal mentor in the Alexander Technique, who,
upon once rather offhandedly remarking to me that I was
"a true intellectual," freed my authentic voice.

and

To Miss Bertha E. Teal (1889–1986)
my high school English teacher in Madrid, Iowa:

Around her classroom walls on hand-lettered banners,
The words of Francis Bacon:

Reading maketh a full man.
Conference maketh a ready man.
Writing maketh an exact man.

Unstinting her effort to instill in us those qualities,
Regardless of individual ability or destiny.

Acknowledgments

I consider this book not only to be a fair representation of
the conceptual dimension of my work as postural educator since 1979, but also—in my choice of epigraphs,
dedications, citations, and allusions—a distinct personal
testament as well. I would like to express appreciation to
John H. M. Austin, M.D., my friend and adviser of 30
years, for his Foreword, to my student Julie Orta for her
personal story, to my longtime editor Phyllis Mueller, to
Dante DeStefano for her perceptive illustrations (pp. 21
and 41–43), and to several colleagues who encouraged my
writing over the years, including Phyllis G. Richmond,
Michael Protzel, and Bruce I. Kodish. Thanks also to
Kathryn Miranda, Lynne T. Shuster, M.D., Gerald Drose,
Ph.D., and Bruce I. Kodish, Ph.D., for back-cover quotes,
and to Jerry Sontag of Mornum Time Press, who deserves
credit for providing, via not one but two readings of my
manuscript, some challenging but ultimately crucial
feedback.

Special thanks to Lorna Rubin of Triad Publishing for
permission to reproduce my Illustrations 2 and 4 from the
late Deborah Caplan's *Back Trouble: A New Approach to
Prevention and Recovery* (Gainesville, FL: Triad Publishing
Company, 1987), to Evelyne Magne of Editions Maloine,
Paris, for gracious assistance in obtaining permission to
reproduce I. A. Kapandji's matchless illustrations in my

Chapter 7, and to George Eckard for the back cover photo.

Finally, to Kimberley Martin and Jera Publishing, LLC, of Roswell, Georgia, for Book Design Wizard 2.0, their excellent book design and layout software, for expert consulting on self-publishing, and—though last, not least—for the very artful cover, by which, in this case, I venture to say, you *can* tell something about the book.

Thanks beyond telling to Dr. Solange Bonnet for both conjugal and material support on my life's journey.

Foreword

"Posture follows movement like a shadow."
Sir Charles Sherrington (1857–1952)

Posture very much has quality ("posturality"), and I am happy to say that this short book genuinely explains both that posture can be improved and how. While Ron Dennis nicely surveys a full range of alternative medicine approaches, the book's viewpoint is mainly that of a truly profound approach: the Alexander Technique—named for its founder, F. Matthias Alexander (1869–1955). Simply put, "Alexander lessons" involve a certified teacher using hands-on guidance to teach awareness of one's movements and posture, thereby allowing the student to choose improved elongation and poise. Ron is an experienced teacher and essayist in this realm.

Posture is an activity of the voluntary muscular system. The term "voluntary" is key here. The Alexander Technique is a valuable—I would say central—way to optimize one's never-ending choices in the use of those muscles.

Scientific validation for the Alexander Technique includes a major British study of 579 patients with chronic or recurrent back pain: Alexander lessons caused long-term decreases in pain and increases in quality of life (P. Little et al., *British Medical Journal*, 2008;337:a884). Also a researcher on the Technique, Ron Dennis has shown that Alexander lessons improved balance in a study of elderly women (*Journal of Gerontology*, 1999;54:M8–11).

The Posturality of the Person is written for everyone, whether a newcomer to the Alexander approach or an experienced student. (A special smile, however, is in order for the experienced student: the title parallels that of *The Use of the Self*, the best-known book by Alexander himself.)

Do not miss reading the appendix by Julie Orta, whose journey was to learn inhibition of unnecessary habitual muscular tensions that had caused her great distress. In truth, practically all of us who have had Alexander lessons can tell a similarly favorable story, even if not necessarily as dramatic as hers.

Ron Dennis is to be commended. This book explains sympathetically and succinctly normal posturality and how its cultivation can indeed improve the quality of one's life.

John H. M. Austin, M.D.
Professor Emeritus of Radiology
Columbia University
February 26, 2012

Table of Contents

1 Introduction

The purpose of this book is to inform you about *posturality*, a crucial aspect of individual and collective human being. Having worked professionally as a teacher in this area for almost 35 years, I am all too aware of the dearth of knowledge, both practical and theoretical, among lay people and professionals, about posturality. My students, most of whom come to me because they are in pain, tell me that they suspect that their posture is somehow connected with their problem, but that they don't know what to do about it.

Often these students have found me only after unsatisfactory experiences with other, more conventional practitioners: orthopedists, chiropractors, and physical and massage therapists. But because I know how to look, almost always I see at once postural factors that are at least contributing to, if not outright causing, the person's symptoms. I am astounded, but not truly surprised, that I, as last consulted, am apparently the first to so see.[1]

---

[1] You might well ask, as did my editor, just how *do* I know how to look? Well, it is basically through a *learning process* similar to that undergone by livestock or animal judges, namely, that of regarding with interest and discernment many, many individuals—as they "live and move and have their being"—relative to a *breed standard*. Only quantifiable in very limited terms, this "breed standard" for human posturality is indeed the subject of this book. For an actual case, see "Appendix I ~Julie O."

This situation most likely prevails because the serious study of posturality, its nature and effects, has long been absent from—truth be told, it was never much present *in*—the required curriculum of healthful living.

Let me be clear about this: it is not that the essential facts are unknown—indeed the literature is vast—but rather that a comprehensive, comprehensible, and workable theory of *normal posturality* has been lacking. This book aims to present that theory together with practical help toward its implementation.

As to the unfamiliar term "posturality," *Webster's New International Dictionary*[2] says that the suffix "-ity" indicates the state or quality of something—mentality, physicality, personality—thus posturality, the state or quality of one's posture. One must go even beyond the current online edition of *Merriam-Webster's Collegiate* to a specialized dictionary of psychology to find "posturality" defined as "the study of postures, used mostly by directors of theatricals in training actors how to demonstrate and portray various emotional states."[3] "Posturology," however, would seem to be the term more accurately so defined.

"Posture" itself eludes precise definition. Webster's gives "a position or attitude of the body or of bodily parts" and

---

[2] Second Edition, Unabridged, 1940.
[3] Raymond J. Corsini, *The Dictionary of Psychology* (Philadelphia: Brunner/Mazel, 1999).

"a characteristic way of bearing one's body, especially the trunk and head." A whole book dedicated to the subject has it as "the position the body assumes in preparation for the next movement."[4] The point in citing these various definitions is that none of them point the way to *normal*, which is by no means *common*, posturality, toward which anyone who is actually hurting and anyone who wishes not to hurt—at least not from musculoskeletal distortions—should be aspiring.[5]

A word about my target audience and writing style: I wrote in what I intended to be rigorous but accessible form and language for those notably but not exclusively of scientific/critical outlook: for general readers, for healthcare professionals, and for those involved in various aspects of complementary and alternative therapeutics, both as providers and consumers. On the one hand, not "Posture for Dummies," but on the other, neither a ponderous tome. Admittedly, however, in general the exposition is quite dense and needs close reading.

Noteworthy in this regard is Chapter 2, "Conceptual Foundations," whose special role in this book needs explanation. Written earlier as an independent piece, these 22 foundational statements aimed then at presenting in the most logical and economical manner the physi-

---

[4] Robert Roaf, *Posture* (London: Academic Press, 1977), p. 1.
[5] You will find my definition of posture as Proposition 1 of Chapter 2, Conceptual Foundations.

ological and developmental issues relevant to the approach to posturality being advocated. In the present work, however—and despite being numbered as a list—these Foundations are not an outline or summary or "analytical table of contents," and you will *not* be reading a systematic amplification of all of those points. Rather, what these 22 propositions actually comprise is a logically ordered series of statements, stripped of non-essentials, to be taken (or not) at face value: a comprehensive if condensed theory of posture and postural education culminating in the concepts of *Length* and *Lengthening* (§§19–22), which in turn form the subjects, for the most part, of the rest of the book. In this respect, the Foundations could be compared to a musical overture, complete in itself but foreshadowing the larger work to follow.

Such concentrated stuff, however, can be challenging to read, as in a mathematical proof, where the relationship between one statement and the next is not always immediately obvious. Or again, like a chain, each link separate and distinct but inextricably connected to both its neighbors. But given the widespread habit of skimming quickly for the gist, as it were, it is easy enough for one to assume that having passed eyes over recognizable words equates to comprehension. *It ain't necessarily so.* Thus, I urge you to pause after each proposition to check your understanding before passing to the next, and to observe the

re-reading suggested in the chapters.[6] I would also suggest that you put a bookmark there at p. 7—now would
be a good time—for easy reference when the time comes.

Indeed, I believe this book to be a guide ultimately to a
higher order of postural understanding and experience,
and that this elevation is a vital aspect of our health,
productivity, and well-being. The part of this journey that
can be made essentially in thought is sufficiently contained, I think, in the Conceptual Foundations through
§18. However, those beginning with §19 dealing with
Length and *Lengthening* derive from not only reflection
but also *experience* on my part. There is thus a dimension
to them unavailable to readers without similar experience. Understanding conceptually the book's successive
materials will not, of course, *provide* this experience—
necessarily *sui generis*—but my hope is that an increase
of knowledge will lead readers to further action and dis-
covery in that direction. In any case, that was a main
intention in writing the book.

Remaining in this introduction is to disclose that my
approach to this subject is by no means original, but in
the main embodies the principles and methods of

---

[6] Some of these propositions may seem obvious, but they were far
from so as I wrote. Recently I encountered a quotation from George
Orwell that fairly said it for me: "To see what is in front of one's nose
needs a constant struggle" (Andrew Sullivan, "The Long Game,"
Newsweek, January 23, 2012, p. 35).

F. Matthias Alexander (1869–1955), founder of the work now known as the Alexander Technique. Myself a teacher of the Technique, I realize that Alexander himself would likely have been less than supportive of my interpretation of his work in such strong and seemingly exclusionary postural terms, an attitude shared by many present-day Alexander teachers. But I also know from long experience that the public that knows about the Technique at all *does* see it primarily in its postural aspect, and, provided that posture is understood as in §1 of the next chapter, I have come over time essentially to concur in that judgment.

2 Conceptual Foundations

§1. Posture comprises the flow through spacetime of all activity of bodily support and movement in the course of living.

§2. The effect of posture as response to gravitational stress on bodily functioning is *constant* (stress as in Mechanics—"an applied force or system of forces that tends to strain or deform a body").

§3. Support and movement do not exist apart from each other in the living person; all support involves movement, all movement involves support.

§4. Neither do body and mind exist apart from each other in the living person; rather, these terms refer to different aspects of *one unified process*. Posture must be viewed inclusively as support-movement, body-mind, or psycho-physical activity.

§5. A comprehensively valid approach to posture must recognize and take into account in its theory and practice this constant, unified, psycho-physical process.

§6. Posture is not fixed from biological inheritance but evolves as a learning process from its genetic and developmental base; posture is a function both of innate factors (reflexes, broadly speaking) and of habit (acquired and more-or-less stereotypical behavior).

§7. Because the innate and the acquired aspects of postural development proceed continuously and simultaneously from birth onwards, only in very general terms can a clear distinction be made in the living person between the two.

§8. Generally, the acquired or habitual aspect of posture develops contingently (by learning) rather than systematically (by training), as a function of the individual's conscious and unconscious responses to the physical, emotional, and cognitive demands of the particular life as actually lived.

§9. To the extent that postural habit is learned, it can through conscious effort be re-learned or modified.

§10. All the foregoing, especially the contingency of postural habit as acquired (§8), imply an issue of quality in the individual's posture, i.e., to what extent this particular posture that has developed is a factor for better or worse in terms of overall functioning.

§11. Where quality is an issue, assessment is relevant; postural quality can be assessed.

§12. Postural quality varies from moment to moment; the assessment of postural quality, whether by an outside observer or by the individual in question, is always conditional relative to the present moment. Assertions about stable postural quality ("I have good/bad posture") are thus undue generalizations, subject to further observation and assessment. "Right now" is the only available time for such assessment.

§13. The assessment of postural quality by an outside observer implies comprehensive knowledge of posture as here delineated combined with experience in applying this knowledge to individual variability.

§14. Ultimately, the assessment of postural quality may be accomplished only by the self-aware individual, through comparing manifest action in real time with a sufficiently valid subjective criterion of postural quality.

§15. Psycho-physically, this criterion is termed "accurate proprioceptive perception."[1]

§16. Accurate proprioceptive perception gives a sense of manifest posture corresponding to the actuality of that

----

[1] Proprioception is "the normal ongoing awareness, mediated by the action of proprioceptors, of the position, balance, and movement of one's own body, or any of its parts"; a proprioceptor is "a receptor [nerve cell that in proprioception responds to stretch, pressure, or displacement] located in muscle, tendon, joint, or vestibular apparatus, whose reflex function is locomotor or postural" (*Blakiston's Pocket Medical Dictionary*, Fourth Edition). *Kinesthesis* (movement sense) is not synonomous with but actually is a subset of proprioception.

posture: disparity between perception and reality can occur because *postural habit conditions postural perception.* For example, the individual with a clearly observable head tilt does not necessarily perceive it as such because visual mechanisms compensate to maintain an upright or "straight" visual field, leading to an unconscious and often-inaccurate postural self-assessment. Many examples of this association between postural habit and proprioceptive perception could be cited; clinical experience indicates that inaccurate proprioceptive perception is not only common but also detrimental to normal functioning in varying degrees among so-called normal as well as symptomatic individuals.

§17. The development of accurate proprioceptive perception is thus the main purpose of postural education.

§18. This educational process provides direct experiences in real time of correct or normal posture: correct experiences condition the individual toward correct and accurate perception.

§19. Posturality is normal when the individual's bodily movement and support are carried out with the skeleton in general and the spine in particular at optimal structural dimension. Minimizing structural stress and preventing strain require that the jointed bodily structure be mechanically well-organized over the base of support. Statically, this organization is usually termed "alignment"; dynamically, there appears to be no descriptive term other than the generic "movement." Both static and dynamic aspects of bodily organization can be incorporated in a practical process called "lengthening."[2]

§20. Conceptually, lengthening means that in standing, sitting, walking, bending, or any activity whatever, one must prevent both unnecessary muscular effort and undue distortions of the natural curves of the spine; full appropriation of lengthening, however, comes only through experience.

§21. Posturality is sub-normal when, through incomplete response to the gravitational challenge and/or unduly contracted musculature, the individual is not lengthening.

§22. "Lengthening" by whatever name is the required principle that unifies the theory of posture as both support and movement. In practice, this principle enables the competent teacher-therapist to assess postural quality reliably and, through the employment of manual and verbal cues and without arbitrary physical exercises, to provide experiences of a normal posturality leading to accurate proprioceptive perception.

---

[2] To the best of my knowledge, the concept of lengthening to characterize the integration of support and movement in human posture was originated by F. Matthias Alexander in his *Constructive Conscious Control of the Individual* and expanded upon in *The Use of the Self* (1923 and 1932, resp., various editions and reprints).

3 Length and Lengthening

Cowboy humorist Will Rogers once said, "Everybody talks about the weather, but nobody ever does anything about it." Just so, everybody knows about posture, but relatively few do anything about it, as much from lack of knowledge and an effective method as from lack of motivation. The problem is that posture and posturality have been much studied but little understood in terms of what constitutes normal posture and how to achieve or, better said, cultivate it. For, like a garden, which is never "achieved," one must rather ongoingly foster the conditions that promote desired growth while minimizing those that interfere with it. The conditions that promote a normal posturality are the practical understandings and actions associated with the concepts of "length" and "lengthening." These are the keys, promised in the Introduction, to a comprehensive theory of postural correction and control.

One aspect of what is meant by "length" (hereafter, Length) is shown by Illustration 1 on the following page:

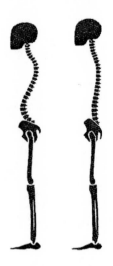

Illustration 1

The spine shown on the left becomes functionally but not structurally longer as it changes to that of its counterpart on the right. This change is what is known in common parlance as "standing up straight," but "straight" is a misleading description of the picture. The spine is still curved but the curves have become less pronounced by the differential action of muscles—some doing less and some doing more—on the spine's structure. It is obvious that this change cannot be effected by a string pulling up on the head, as popular advice counsels. It also is important to begin to realize that images and "tips" for the improvement of posture based on misleading models or analogies have the potential of leading to wrong actions in the attempt to carry them out—I have seen many over-straightened necks as a result of such misplaced zeal. A more appropriate image for the Lengthening in Illustration 1 would be that of inflating a tire gone low, but in truth no image is required once the principle is understood.

Illustration 2 shows functionally shortened and lengthened spines in sitting:

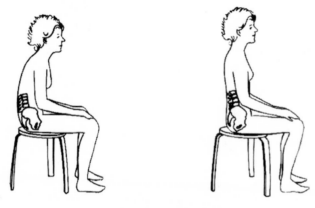

Illustration 2

In your mind's eye visualize the movement that takes place from the one to the other, in either direction for that matter. Better yet, actually try it! Now, re-read §1 of "Conceptual Foundations," my definition of posture. (Hereafter, when referring you to "Conceptual Foundations," I will use only the § symbol.) More and more, begin to think of posture as a flow through space and time, rather than as static positions assumed for special activities. The idea of Length, combined with that of Flow, is the dynamic concept that yields a workable theory of normal posturality. Not a special way of doing certain things, but a specific way of doing all things. That specific way is Lengthening. Our postural mantra should be, "More and more, I Flow with Length."

Because of its many vertebrae and its supportive function vis-a-vis upright posture, the spine is the most common and also the most important bodily structure liable to compromises of Length, but shortening may occur at any joint in the body's weight-bearing chain where muscular activity does not keep structures aligned in the direction of required support. Illustration 3 shows this kind of situation at the left foot-ankle joint (viewed from behind):

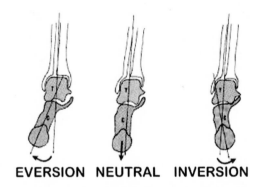

EVERSION NEUTRAL INVERSION

From *Foot and Ankle Pain, Second Edition,* Cailliet, Rene,1968, page 10, F. A. Davis Company, Philadelphia, PA 19103, with permission.

Illustration 3

In *eversion,* Length is lost in one direction (on the outside), and in *inversion* the other. Strikingly illustrated here is how Length is a function of a specific distribution of muscular activity. In eversion, muscles on the inside of the joint (toward the midline of the body) are not contracting strongly enough, while in inversion, it is the muscles on the outside. Also to realize is that these apparently small—as little as an eighth-inch—distortions in joint alignment are located near the very bottom of the bodily weight-bearing chain, with unequal pressures on the joint surfaces. Some people experience these differential pressures as pain. In general, we should maintain a provisional attitude about apparently small distortions in posture. We can't really assess how such distortions are affecting bodily function and comfort until we become aware of and begin to do something about them.

Illustration 4 shows the crucial postural relationship between head and neck (or more accurately, head and spine—in the world of muscles, nerves, and bones there are no "necks," the term conveniently but sometimes misleadingly labeling that part of the spine between the top of the rib cage and the head):

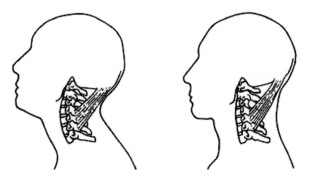

Illustration 4

On the left, the musculature joining head to spine is shortened, either pulling the head or allowing it to fall into this position on the spine. This postural syndrome, which has the distinct possibility of over-approximating the cervical bones (stenosis) is widespread among civilized people, and may derive, at least in part, from chronic anxiety.[1] On the right, the muscles have released into Length, allowing the head to sit squarely atop the spine and giving the bones and discs adequate space.

In terms of overall postural coordination, the cervical musculature is extremely rich in muscle spindles, microscopic neural structures within the muscles that are responsive to stretch and that control the reflex maintenance of balance. Chronic shortening and tension in this musculature, a potential source of discomfort in and of itself, can also produce "static" on what should be clear controlling signals within the nervous system.[2]

Also to be noted is the effect of shortening on the posture of the eyes: because the head is chronically tilted back, the eyes must be held in slight counter-clockwise rotation in order to see directly ahead. If the head posture changes toward that of the right side of Illustration 4, the gaze will

---

[1] This is my hypothesis as suggested by Frank Pierce Jones' investigation of the startle pattern in *Body Awareness in Action* (New York: Schocken Books, 1976), pp. 131–133.

[2] George B. Whatmore and Daniel R. Kohli, "Dysponesis: A Neurophysiologic Factor in Functional Disorders," *Behavioral Science* (Vol. 13, March 1968), pp. 102–124.

be directed downward because the eyes do not immediately and automatically change their habitual posture relative to that of the head. A person correcting a "back-and-down" head posture (Illustration 4, left diagram) will need to allow the eyes to adjust to a different level as well. This kind of observation illustrates the postural interconnectedness that must be taken into account in any program of postural education or therapy.

Although by no means comprehensive, this chapter has aimed to acquaint you with the essential "what" of Length and Lengthening. Succeeding chapters will address both the "why" and the "how." Knowing these broad principles will take you further, should you decide to go, than either piecemeal "tips" or special exercises and manipulations of all types that are based on incomplete understanding and/or debatable values.[3] For now, please go back and re-read §§19–22, which hopefully will be more clear.

_____

[3] A debatable value, for example, is that of "flexibility of the spine." As will be discussed in Chapter 6, bending of the spine in the name of "flexibility," without a reasonably clear specification of how much or in what manner, can lead to serious problems.

4 *Why* Lengthen?

Why indeed *should* we Lengthen?

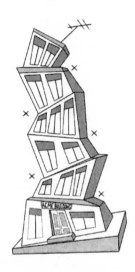

Illustration 5

Honestly, need I say much more? It doesn't take an engineering degree to see that the mechanical strains produced by gravitational force on the building, not only at the Xs but throughout, result from the load's not being supported in the most direct path to the ground. Truth be told, if we erected our buildings as sloppily as many us erect our bodies, the landscape would be littered with ruins!

Illustration 5 is directly analogous to the left figure of Illustration 1 (p. 14), a difference being that bodies can compensate for structural distortion by muscular action, where buildings can't. In bodies, muscles reflexively take up the work of stabilizing the structure, but the strain remains, which is why bodies usually hurt before they collapse, as the 80% of people who either have or will experience significant back pain can readily attest.[1] Thus, a main reason why we should Lengthen is to reduce structural strain in the task of carrying our weight on Mother Earth. In our bodies, muscles not only move bones but position bones relative to each other so as to provide a stable path to the ground. In the shortened body, where weight-bearing joints are in faulty alignment, muscular action must take up a disproportionate share of this stabilizing function, resulting not only in fatigue but also in abnormal pressures within the joints and on nerves. As J. E. Goldthwait, M.D., an early 20th-century physician and one-time president of the American Ortho-pedic Association, succinctly put it:

> An individual is in the best health only when the body is so used that there is no strain on any of its parts. This means that, when standing, the body is held fully erect, with no strain on the joints, the bones, the ligaments, the muscles or any other structure.[2]

A "fully erect" standing body is a Lengthened body, as we saw in Chapter 2. It is also a walking, sitting, folding,

---

[1] *MedlinePlus*, (n.d.) *Back Pain.* Retrieved from http://www.nlm.nih.gov/medlineplus/backpain.html.
[2] Joel E. Goldthwait et al., *Essentials of Body Mechanics in Health and Disease*, Fifth Ed. (Philadelphia: Lippincott, 1952), p. 1.

speaking, and limb-using body, which we will learn more about in Chapter 4.

Goldthwait continued the above observation with the second main reason for Lengthening:

> There should be adequate room for all the viscera, so that their function can be performed normally unless there be some congenital defect.

Illustrations 6 and 7 deserve full attention because they illuminate not only the current point about space for the viscera (internal organs) but several others as well:

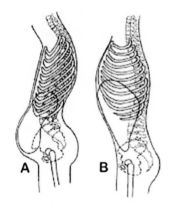

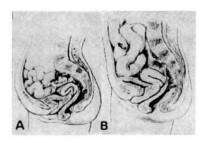

Illustration 6   *Illustration 7*

From *Essentials of Body Mechanics in Health and Disease,* Joel E. Goldthwait et al., Fifth Edition, 1952, pp. 64, 174, J. B. Lippincott Company, Philadelphia, PA 19103, with permission.

There is so much to say about these diagrams it is hard to know where to start—you should study them until you have fully integrated the images with the text.

Illustration 6A shows the shortening consequences of insufficient action of the "abominable" muscles. The viscera, collectively represented by the bean-shaped line—the "bag," as I call it for short—drop down and forward, distorting the spine by exaggerating its curves. The rib cage and its occupants, the heart and lungs, are depressed and reduced in capacity, and the viscera sag down into the pelvis. In dramatic contrast, Illustration 6B (admittedly somewhat over-drawn for emphasis) shows a Lengthened and optimally supportive spine, as well as abdominal muscles (especially the lower ones, more on that later) powerfully pushing the visceral "bag" back and up into the torso, stabilizing the spine and restoring an appropriate lumbar curve while lifting and expanding the rib cage. Read and look, look and read, until you can see in your mind's eye the movement from 6A to 6B and begin to have a "feel" for the forces and displacements involved.

Know that, as 70% or so water, the visceral contents are essentially non-compressible. They are thus moved hydraulically as a unit, like the brakes in your car, by contraction of the abdominals, and the force of this contraction is transmitted undiminished up through the torso and all the way out the head. Talk about exercise! The visceral organs, including fat but not muscle tissue, weigh about 17 to 23% of body mass in adult males and females, respectively.[3] In a 128-lb. adult female, for example, the visceral weight would thus be just a little over 29 lbs. Moving that amount of weight 2" back and up in the body would be almost half again as much work than lifting two 10 lb. dumbbells 2" off the floor—not a huge lift but, in the case of the abdominals, one that is potentially going on continuously except while reclining. Talk about Lengthening! This muscular action and coordination of the abdominals is *and should be clearly understood as* the veritable keystone of postural support in the body!

Illustration 7 gets literally to the "guts" of the story, and what a story it is. Diagrammed are a female pelvis and viscera, but the same observations would apply to a male as well, *mutatis mutandis* as Latin has it ("the necessary [!] changes being made"). In 6A and 7A we see how, when the abdominal muscles aren't doing their job, the intestines fall into the basement, as it were, pressing on and otherwise affecting the plumbing—in the female, bladder and uterus primarily, while in the male, bladder and prostate.

In 6B and 7B, with the abdominals correctly activated, the intestines are pushed back and up to give the pelvic

---

[3] These figures are based upon data in Table 2, "Weight distribution of organs and tissues," Sheng, Hwai-Ping, "Body Composition," *Encyclopedia of Food and Culture* (New York: Charles Scribner's Sons, 2003). Visceral fat was conservatively estimated as half of total adipose tissue.

organs the space they need to function properly. Think about this the next time you hear or see a commercial touting relief for incontinence, prostate problems, or "female complaints," as they used to say. Also think about the general biological principle that pressure is destructive of tissue. With those things in mind, perhaps the "why" of Lengthening may acquire a relevance beyond that of back pain, neck pain, and musculoskeletal pains in general, not that those are trivial matters by any means.

Not a bad idea to read Conceptual Foundations again—at least look at §2, which should be much clearer now.

5 Good Grief, How *Do* I Lengthen Anyway?

A word of disclaimer here: this is not a "how-to" book.[1]
Skill learning of any kind—and normal posturality is
indeed a skill—involves many variables, and most people
are well-advised to seek professional help, as they often
do more or less readily when learning golf, guitar, tango,
or any other of the myriad skills they wish to acquire.

Why then a chapter on how to Lengthen? One reason is to
give some practical if incomplete guidance for your own
exploration. (That's why you're reading this book, right?)
A second reason is to furnish a map of the territory,
showing the main routes, features of interest, and possible detours or dead ends.[2] And a third is to help you
evaluate any professional help that you might seek out:
there are many purveyors of postural education and
therapy—the Alexander Technique, yoga, Pilates, chiropractors, physical therapists, to name a few—but not all
of them are equally qualified or effective. Before investing
your time and treasure—your body, too—use the knowledge gained from this book to determine whether poten-

---

[1] Especially is this so regarding the relief of what is often called
"muscular tension." Please see Appendix III, "Muscles and Mentals:
Why We Get Tense," for an appreciation of this aspect of posturality.
[2] The analogy of a physical map to a verbal one (or to any other form
of representation) is a key concept of Alfred Korzybski's *general
semantics*, with which every language-using person should be familiar—see Chapter 9, "Bibliographic Essay."

tial providers both have and practice a credible theory on which to base their instruction.

Now I'll invite you to join a little scenario with me called The Wilted Plant. You probably have had the experience of forgetting to water a plant—you come into the room and see it all wilted and droopy. You dash off for your watering can and give the plant a good drink, fervently hoping that you caught it in time. Having done all you could do, you go about your life, to return perhaps a half-hour later to see how your ailing friend is doing. Well, if indeed you caught it in time, it is back to its old self, stems and leaves full of the life-restoring fluid that came in through the roots and up through the plant's vascular system. Your plant did not "stand up straight," it Lengthened. Water, moving up to fill it, restored it to its natural fullness of dimension and vigor.

Your turn. From standing, let yourself wilt into a good slump. (You may be quite skilled at this already.) Let your head drop back onto your neck (oops, spine), and let your whole body droop downward—spine, hips, knees, ankles. Now, gently, as if water were quietly flowing up through your bones and joints (but of course it's muscular action), begin to move up through your ankles, your knees, your hips, your spine, and all the way up, 'til your head is just sitting on this column of gently up-flowing energy. Take about 10 seconds to enact this scenario.

Done? Then I will tell you, as I tell my students, "Guess what, you didn't stand up straight, you Lengthened." But it doesn't matter, if you moved from a slump gently upward through your body until you couldn't go further without straining, you Lengthened. Your technique may be less than perfect, your end result not what it might be with coaching, but nevertheless, you Lengthened. You can re-enact this little scenario (notice I didn't say, "Do this exercise," which is often the route to mindless repetition) any time you remember it. If you're at a cocktail party and don't wish to appear odd, just do a teeny wilt and Lengthen out of it!

Now we'll experiment with Lengthening from the other direction. Stand in a position of what in the military is called a "brace," the exaggerated form of the standard position of Attention—head up, chin tucked, shoulders back, thumbs facing forward, etc. Brace as tightly as you can without hurting yourself. Illustration 8, from a 19th-century book extolling "Swedish educational gymnastics," shows this position:[3]

---

[3] Hartvig Nissen, *A B C of the Swedish System of Educational Gymnastics* (Boston: Educational Publishing Co., 1892), p. 7.

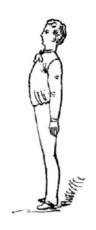

Illustration 8

Take a little break from your brace and think with me for a moment. Can you see that, compared with a slump, where you're shortened in front, in a brace, you're shortened in back? Tight and narrowed between the shoulder blades and in the small of your back? Also that, where a slump results from too little activity in the muscles of the back, a brace results from too much?

Now go back to your tightly held brace and begin, like an over-inflated tire, to let the air out of it, so to speak: let your chest soften downward as you release your tight neck and shoulders and let your back release out of its grip as well. Keep going until you get all the way into a slump, pause there a moment, and then ease yourself back up into Length—not "up tight," but "up released." As I said before, your technique may be less than perfect, your end result not be what it might with coaching, but nevertheless, you Lengthened. Now you can begin both conceptually to appreciate and actually to experience how a normal posturality is poised delicately between a slump and a brace.

Pausing and Organizing[4]

In working through the above scenarios with any degree of care and attention, you are implicitly employing two processes that are mostly absent in habitual activity: you are *pausing*—even if barely—as you go along, in order to think what comes next, and you are *organizing*—even if unsurely—your actions to comply with your thinking. This process of pausing and organizing at the conscious level is what characterizes true Practice (with a capital "P"), as opposed to small-p practice, which is often just mindless repetition.

Now think a little deeper into this with me. Let's say there's something you wish to do better, your golf swing, for example. Going about this, you get some ideas—by reading or watching, or maybe from a teacher, and then you begin to practice—pausing and organizing as you prepare and perform the swing's movement. Usually you will experience improvement over time in terms of the accuracy and distance of your strokes, because accuracy and distance are clear and quantifiable criteria of performance.

---

[4] Inhibition and Direction for readers familiar with the Alexander Technique.

In the case of Lengthening (the subject of this chapter, remember?), the situation is very different because its criteria—whether you're really changing or not—are not clear and quantifiable like those of many acquired skills. Take a minute to re-read §12. Because postural quality—Length—varies from moment to moment, the only time it can be experienced as improved is in the conscious moment of attending to it. This means that in those countless other moments, we really don't know whether it's different or not.

Does this mean that we have to think about Lengthening every moment? Fortunately not, since that would be impossible in any case—awareness has many more jobs than just paying attention to posture. But, in the same way that our very first halting but determined attempts as infants to learn to carry ourselves upright became reliable habit with practice over time, we may be confident, based on the experience of your author and many other people who have followed this path, that the same process, aided by conscious awareness and intention, is taking place as we Pause and Organize—again Pause and Organize—yet again Pause and Organize—in moving ourselves through the actions and days that constitute our life. Bear in mind, as you go along, this observation from Professor N. (Nikolai) Bernstein, a great Russian physiologist and the father of modern movement science:

> The motor activity of organisms is of enormous biological significance—it is practically the only way in which the or-

ganism not only interacts with the surrounding environment, but actively alters this environment, altering it with
respect to particular results.[5]

The next chapter will discuss how we take a Lengthened
posturality into those enormously significant doings
through which we actually live our days.

---

[5] N. Bernstein, *The Co-ordination and Regulation of Movements*
(Oxford: Pergamon Press, 1967), p. 114.

6 Dynamic Posturality ~ Moving with Length

Generally, we tend to assume that "posture" refers essentially to static positions, and that "movement" likewise refers to—well, what else but movements? Now is precisely the time to re-read §3 (please do it now) and to begin to understand it more fully. For this we turn to a lengthy but necessary quotation from a leading authority, physiologist Tristan D. M. Roberts of the University of Glasgow. In the first paragraph of the first chapter of his massive *Neurophysiology of Postural Mechanisms* (415 small-print pages) Roberts says:

> A movement may be thought of as a change in posture. Alternatively, one might be tempted to regard the voluntary movements of the hands in man as something different from the posture of the rest of the body, so that "posture" and "movement" could be dealt with separately. However, even such small movements of the fingers as occur in writing, commonly involve adjustments in the activity of the muscles of the arm, and often there are accompanying head movements also as the eyes follow the task in hand. These adjustments of the head and arms alter the disposition of the weight of the body in relation to the supports, so that muscles in many different parts of the body become involved, as, for example, in the other arm, or in the legs and trunk. All this background activity needs to be accurately co-ordinated for the successful performance of the desired movement of the fingers. *There is no difficulty in regarding*

the background activity as "postural" [my italics]. According-
ly, because this background activity is essential to the successful performance of the voluntary movement itself and
has to be co-ordinated with it, *there are advantages in treating the whole process as a unity* [my italics].[1]

Roberts here is telling us that in the neuro-musculo-
skeletal reality of our bodies, there are no such things as
"posture" and "movement": these are abstract concepts
pointing to aspects of one unified process, but not real
things in themselves. The practical significance of this
insight is that our efforts in the direction of postural
control and correction need to be based in procedures
that recognize and take into account this truth. Our work
in this chapter, then, is to better understand this Dynamic Posturality—in terms of this book's thesis, how do we
Lengthen even as we move?

To put the matter in the smallest of nutshells, if we will
fold at the right places and *not bend* at the wrong ones as
we perform the movements that make up the actions of
our daily lives, then we will be going a long way toward
Lengthening in Dynamic Posturality.

Before going into this pronunciamento more fully, think
with me for a bit about what I call Modes of Existential
Movement (MEMs). They are "existential" not in the philo-
sophical sense, but rather as pointing to main ways in

---

[1] Second Edition (London: Butterworths, 1978), p. 9.

which we all must move just in existing through a day, regardless of those actions required for specialized skills:

1. *Standing*;
2. Transporting ourselves across the world, commonly called *Walking* (or occasionally Running);
3. Going toward and away from the ground over a stationary base, commonly called Bending, but better understood as *Folding*;
4. Sustaining a more-or-less erect posture with one's bottom on a more-or-less stable platform of some sort, namely *Sitting*;
5. *Limbing*, that is, using limbs and their extensions (fingers and toes), especially the arms in Reaching, as in, for example, combing the hair, typing, or raking, but also the legs as in Jumping;
6. Managing breath and vocal apparatus in *Speaking*;
7. Various activities, active and passive, taking place in *Lying* (reclining).

Of course, these seven MEMs aren't mutually exclusive—we can walk while we talk, etc.—and always involve transitions one to the next. But at least the seven-fold schema gives a conceptual framework for reflecting on things that would ordinarily never rise to consciousness.[2]

---

[2] *Breathing* is not included in this classification because it is the usually reflexive and unconscious accompaniment to the voluntary actions of Existential Movement; existentially I don't "breathe down," I "sit down." Chapter 7 is devoted entirely to breath in both its reflexive and voluntary aspects.

Revenons à nos moutons, as the French say—"Let's get back to our sheep." The "folding at the right places" alluded to above (p. 36) takes place in MEM 3 at the hips, knees, and ankles, and additionally at the forefoot in MEM 2. The "not bending at the wrong places" takes place with all MEMs mainly in the spine. This last requires further explanation, and I hope you will bear with the somewhat meandering nature of this exposition, but it is unavoidable because verbal discourse is a linear process—a melody, as it were—while our posturality goes on all at once—chords in progression, so to speak—thus precluding a strictly by-the-numbers account, inconsistent with the nature of the beast, so we must meander to get anywhere at all.

So, *revenons à nos moutons*. While the spine by virtue of its composition of many bones (vertebrae) connected by cartilaginous structures (intervertebral discs) is a structure fully compatible with both support and movement in normal human activity, it really does not much like to be bent—particularly in the "rounded back" attitude of flexion—and especially over long periods and under conditions of load. Under such conditions, if the spine is held bent out of its normal shape, the relatively soft discs tend to be pushed out from their normal snug position between the vertebral bodies and back toward the sensitive nerve rootlets of the spinal cord that emerge on both sides between each pair of vertebrae. Discs pushed too far in this direction impinge on these nerves, which in their turn don't much like the abnormal pressure of errant discs, and their protest—in addition to the warning signal of pain—often takes the form of messages to Control Central (the Central Nervous System) to stop the system from further movement in that direction (which is the function of muscular locking or spasm) by means of which the system is actually doing its best to relieve that d--- pressure, but not without cost in terms of pain or immobility to the person undergoing it! A further complication is that the fibrous outer rings of the discs, having no blood supply and hence tending to dry with aging, and being prone as well to developing cracks and tears from life's traumas large and small, become structurally compromised, making them even more liable to displacement, the so-called "ruptured disc" when severe (Illustration 9).

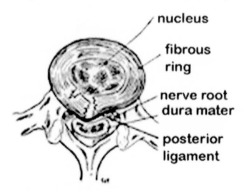

From *The Slipped Disk, Third Edition,* Cyriax, James, 1980, p. 8, Charles Scribner's Sons, New York, NY, with permission.

Illustration 9

So there you have the essential scenario of much posturally induced spinal pain: pressure on spinal nerves by structurally compromised discs pushed out of place by excessive spinal bending. The eminent British orthopedist

James Cyriax (d. 1985) pioneered precisely this hypothesis in advocating proper posture in daily movement activities as the therapy-of-choice for typical back problems, as opposed to common "back exercises," which often actually increase undue effort and strain, especially when, as likely, they are performed incorrectly.[3]

The following series of illustrations shows how the principles of Lengthening and Folding find application in various Modes of Existential Movement as presented in this chapter. Obviously such snapshots, illustrative but necessarily static, can't capture the full sweep of actual movements—it's up to your agile imagination to supply that.

---

[3] James Cyriax, M.D., *The Slipped Disc* (New York: Scribner's, 1980), *passim* and esp. Chapter 7, "Posture vs. Exercises."

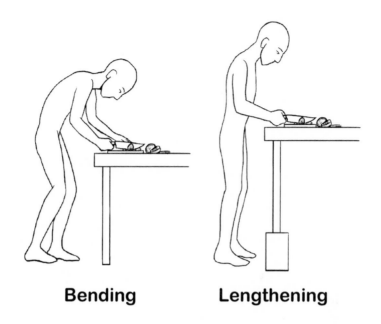

Bending   **Lengthening**

Standing at desk or table

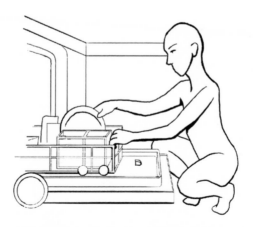

Folding and Lengthening

Loading/unloading dishwasher

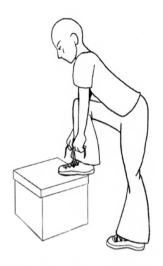

Folding and Lengthening

Tying shoes

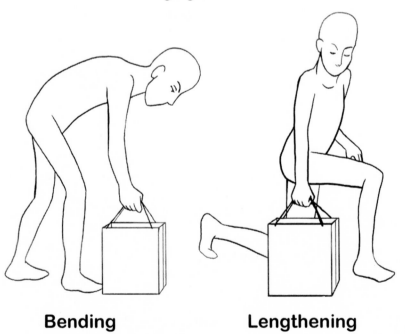

Bending　　　　　**Lengthening**

Folding to lift bag

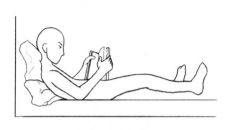 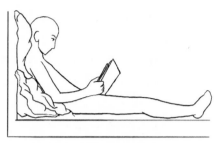

Bending   **Lengthening**

Reading in bed

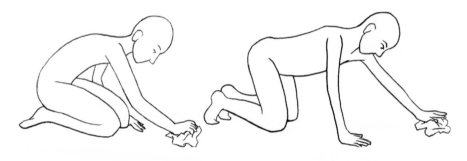

Bending   **Lengthening**

Scrubbing or gardening

How better to close this chapter than with a quotation from the all-but-forgotten source after which it is titled, the article "Dynamic Posture," written by an astute New York physician, one Beckett Howorth, M.D., and published in the *Journal of the American Medical Association* of August 24th, 1946:

Posture has long been thought of in terms of standing and sitting, and correct posture as the erect position assumed when one is under inspection, but posture should really be considered as *the sum total of the positions and movements of the body throughout the day and throughout life* [my italics]. It should include not only the fundamental static positions in lying, sitting and standing, and the variations of these positions but also the dynamic postures of the body in motion or in action, for *it is here that posture becomes most important and most effective* [my italics].[4]

Bravo, Dr. Howorth!

---

[4]p. 1398.

7 Breath As Postural Process

As announced in §1, "Posture comprises the flow through space and time of all activity of bodily support and movement in the course of living." My work would certainly be incomplete without an exposition of how each of us effects, through postural action, the essential gaseous exchange of oxygen and carbon dioxide in our bodies, commonly called "breathing."

I approach the task with misgiving because, even though I have deeply (so to speak) studied breathing over many years, I also realize the difficulty—ultimately, the impossibility—of putting into linear words a process that takes place not only in three-dimensional space but also in the fourth dimension of time. Nevertheless, I must try because 1) the subject is so important, 2) it is so little understood, and 3) there is so much misleading writing and teaching about it. Truth be told, you would need to look long and hard to find a source equal in both scope and brevity to that you are about to read—a veritable Martini, concentrated and powerful, of respiratory lore. Here I hope to reveal for you the Optimal Metabolic Breath, "metabolic" referring to the entire complex of physical and chemical processes that maintain life.

Let's begin by understanding that "breathing" isn't a specialized skill that we need to acquire through rote practice or exercises, like typing. In fact, "breathing," like "neck" (p. 17), isn't a something at all, other than a *label* for the psycho-physical process in which certain actions and reactions, both muscular and chemical, result in the necessary exchange of gases in metabolism.[1] Hardly a trivial distinction, among other things this means that you shouldn't be trying to "breathe correctly" according to some or other dogmatic formula—"breathe from your diaphragm," for example—but rather that you are much better served by coming to understand, in order productively to manage, the postural pattern that results in optimal respiration.

The case actually is that when we truly Lengthen, everything takes place as it should! But with four chapters already on Lengthening, what more can be said? That little word "truly" is the Devil wherein the details now to be gleaned lie.

Look at this picture (Illustration 6, reversed):

---

[1] In the interest of communication, however, and sheerly out of habit, I often use "breathing" as a substantive, reminding myself that I am referring to a verbal label and not a discrete physical thing.

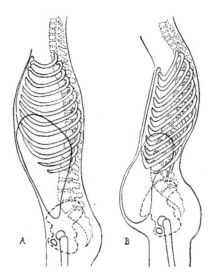

In which rib cage do you think your lungs (and heart, too) would be happier to live? If A is the obvious answer, the next question is, how does rib cage A get that full, expansive shape? A little study will help you see that it is the action of the abdominal muscles that moves the viscera (the "bag," p. 24) as a unit, and that the direction of movement is back toward the spine and also up toward the head. (Actually the movement is also down, but since the bony pelvis blocks the way, the main displacement is up.) This hydraulic action (the viscera are 70% or so water and thus, essentially, non-compressible) pushes up on the diaphragm, which goes all the way round the bottom of the rib cage and domes up into it (think of a contraceptive diaphragm, in terms of its properties of encirclement, containment, and mobility), and thus the rib cage is pushed up from below by the viscera as moved by abdominals as well as held up from the back by the spine.

Our next project is more fully to understand the abdominal musculature. From the inside outward, there are four distinct layers, shown in Illustration 9 :

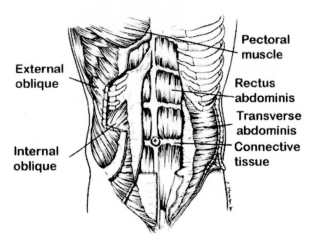

Illustration 9

The innermost layer (transverse abdominis) runs mostly crosswise or transversely, the second and third (internal and external obliques), run slantwise in complementary directions, while the fourth (rectus abdominis) runs vertically from the pubis to the lower rib cage. These four layers of muscle act for the most part synergistically, which means that even though each has its own nerve supply, and thus the capacity for separate activation, they work essentially as a team in the same directions, depending on the support and/or movement required, rather than antagonistically to produce a change in movement direction, as in flexing the bicep, for example.

It is the fourth or top layer, the two recti abdominis, that most concerns us in terms of our postural model and therefore of our consciously organized postural behavior. Notice that structurally the two recti abdominis are not a single muscle on each side, but rather, because of the intervening connective tissue (all-white on the diagram), form two "stacks" of four segments each. Notice also that the lowest segment, running from pubis to just below the navel, is much longer than the others. Now, it's most important to know that each of these segments (eight altogether on both sides) has a separate nerve supply from the spinal cord, meaning that we have the potential for differential control of these muscles (accounting, among other things, for some of the intriguing movements of exotic dancing). In terms of our more prosaic postural model, however, the main implication of this arrangement is that we can control the lower abdominal musculature separately from the upper; it is distinctly possible, and as we will see, definitely desirable, to maintain supportive muscle tone in the lower segments (pubis to navel) while allowing the upper segments to release and lengthen, in both the inflow and the outflow of breath. This is the essential feature of the postural model that both provides support for the spine (which certainly needs it) and also allows movement of the rib cage, where the lungs live.

In questioning students over the years about how they think we breathe, I've learned that often enough they believe that, when we breathe in, the inspired air inflates the lungs and moves the ribs. Actually it is the reverse: we either raise the ribs or lower the diaphragm or both, which increases the internal volume of the thorax, which lowers the pressure, which causes air from outside the body at higher pressure to flow into the internal area of lower pressure, thus "taking a breath."

Now we need to see how this movement of the rib cage is produced, probably the most difficult aspect of our model to visualize and really "get." When you have contemplated the three two-dimensional images of Illustration 10 sufficiently to model them in your mind—first in the three spatial dimensions and then in time—you will have reached a point where you, with Paul the Apostle, no longer "see through a glass darkly," but rather in the full light of understanding—as Hamlet soliloquized, "a consummation devoutly to be wished"!

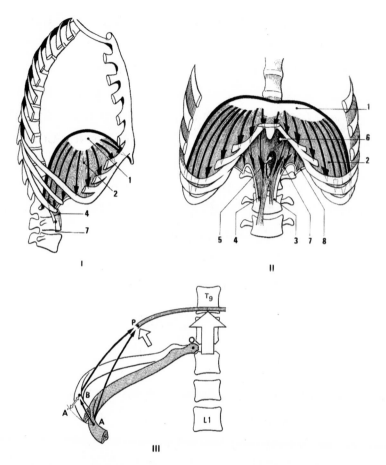

From *The Physiology of the Joints, Vol. 3, Second Ed.,*
Kapandji, I. A., 1974, page 147, Churchill Livingstone,
Edinburgh London and New York, with permission.

Illustration 10

Diagrams I and II of Illustration 10 basically show the
anatomical features of the diaphragm as it attaches to
and is positioned in the rib cage (disregard all of the
arabic numerals and refer only to I, II, and III). To note is
that the diaphragm domes up inside the rib cage, and

that the top of the dome (in white) is not muscular but tendinous—connective not contractile tissue. Also that muscle fibers connect the dome with the lower ribs, and additionally to the spine in back.[2] Of course the area under the diaphragm isn't empty as in the diagram, but rather full of viscera—the "bag." While ostensibly too obvious even to point out, this aspect of structure is often omitted in accounts of respiratory mechanics,[3] but indeed is crucial to understanding how the rib cage is moved by a definite resolution of forces within the body. It is Diagram III that shows in schematic form the muscular actions that produce this resolution of forces.

Look at Diagram III as if the shaded rib were the beginning of an inbreath. The diaphragm contracts, meaning that the muscle fibers that connect it to the lower ribs shorten (schematically Segment A-P). Since the distance between A and P is shortening through muscle contraction, the rib is pulled laterally from A through an arc to A', and also, because of the pivoting action of the rib's attachment to the spine, upwardly to B. And, because the entire rib cage is structurally connected, the displacement illustrated by A to B in the diagram actually represents a

---

[2] These anatomical facts contrast sharply with the naive concept I held as a young clarinetist, namely, that the diaphragm was a flat muscle running straight across the middle of my body which more-or-less flapped in the breeze of breathing.
[3] For example, *Science of Breath: A Practical Guide.* Swami Rama, Rudolph Ballentine, M.D., Alan Hymes, M.D. (Honesdale, PA: Himalayan International Institute of Yoga, Science and Philosophy, 1979).

total movement of the rib cage "out and up." Illustration 11 gives a sidewise view of this total movement (starting on the inbreath from C and moving to C' and corresponding points), clearly showing the "forward" component as well (that is, if undue muscular tensions are not distorting this movement).

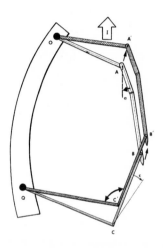

From *The Physiology of the Joints, Vol. 3, Second Ed.,* Kapandji, I. A., 1974, page 143, Churchill Livingstone, Edinburgh London and New York, with permission.

Illustration 11

The foregoing represents a kinematic[4] analysis of rib cage movement. We must now proceed to an understanding of the kinetics involved—movements don't just happen without forces to produce them! Look again at Illustration

---

[4] "Kinematics" refers to spatial displacement in movements regardless of the forces producing them; "kinetics" refers to the actual forces. For example, from the movement standpoint, a movie is a purely kinematic presentation.

10, Diagram III. That mysterious white arrow under the diaphragm represents a directional force, like a vector in a classical physics diagram (excepting that here the magnitude of the force is not-to-scale). So we are meant to see that there is a force acting upward on the diaphragm and that it is coming from below, but, at least from this diagram, we have no clue about what is producing it. Please look again at the illustration on page 47. There we see that the abdominal musculature in B is relaxed, allowing the viscera to drop down and forward, while in A it is energized, pushing the viscera back and up. It is this contraction of the abdominal muscles, as transmitted through the viscera, that produces the force represented by the white arrow. If this upward force is sufficient to keep the dome of the contracting diaphragm relatively high on the inbreath, then, instead of the diaphragm's descending (flattening) as it contracts, and pushing the viscera down and forward, it remains high and, over the fulcrum of the underlying viscera, lifts—picks right up— the rib cage. Don't be discouraged if at first you don't see this: it is as much a skilled accomplishment—requiring practice over time—to form and hold this four dimensional model in the mind as it is to manifest it in the body.

In the foregoing analyis, I've alluded to the structural division of the abdominal musculature into upper and lower. Now it's time to see the functional significance of this structural arrangement. We saw above how each of the eight segments of the two recti abdominis muscles has a separate nerve supply, meaning that with each is the possibility of differential control. Functionally speaking, if the lower segments remain energized (skillfully contracted) during the respiratory cycle, and the upper segments are allowed to release and lengthen, then both high support of the diaphragm and also movement of the rib cage are optimized. Contrariwise, if this musculature is tightly held, top to bottom—as in "suck in your gut"—then the upward movement of the rib cage is curtailed—think of the guys (ropes) holding a tent down—and the resulting tension of competing muscular actions—the diaphragm pulling up and the recti abdominis pulling down—not only compromises efficient respiration but, in extreme cases, can lead to physical and emotional discomfort. Try it for yourself: suck in your gut and hold it while taking a few breaths; I would be surprised if you didn't find it decidedly uncomfortable. No wonder strong men faint while maintaining the military position of Attention!

Contrasted with this model of Breath as Postural Process is the one commonly called Breathe from Your Diaphragm—the ubiquitous directive given to singers, wind players, actors, glass-blowers, etc., not to mention the ordinary person who has enrolled in an exercise class. In terms of practical instruction on this less-than-explicit directive, the student is generally advised to relax the belly on the inbreath, so as to avoid the shallowness and tensions often associated with the dreaded "chest breathing." Illustration 12 gives quite a clear picture of this process by means of a simple mechanical model:

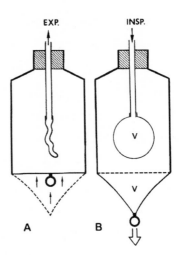

From *The Physiology of the Joints, Vol. 3, Second Ed.,*
Kapandji, I. A., 1974, page 153, Churchill Livingstone,
Edinburgh London and New York, with permission.

Illustration 12

Here we see a bell jar fitted with a rubber diaphragm
stretched across the bottom, a ring attached to the diaphragm for pulling it down, a glass inlet tube to which is
fitted a small rubber balloon, and a stopper through
which the tube passes. Timewise, Diagram A represents
both the end of an expiration (EXP.) and beginning of an
inspiration (INSP.), and Diagram B the end of an inspiration. We are meant to understand that, as the diaphragm
is pulled down from its starting place in Diagram A
(inbreath), the volume of the enclosed space (V in Diagram B) increases by the amount of diaphragmatic displacement, hence the pressure falls and air moves from
the area of higher pressure outside into that of lower
pressure inside, hence inflating the balloon (lungs)

56

attached to the inlet tube, as in Diagram B, quite a fair illustration of the "breathe from your diaphragm" model.

Allow me to question you socratically: "What's wrong with this model? What in it doesn't correspond to the actual anatomical facts that we've discussed?" Yes, the "diaphragm" closes the bottom of the "rib cage" and yes the physics are correct, *but* (and it's a *big but*, pardon the expression), a bell jar is rigid and a real rib cage moves! A real rib cage moves out, up, and forward as powered by the diaphragm as discussed earlier with Illustrations 10 and 11. *The lungs live in the rib cage!* Why would one choose to restrict their vital functions by a type of coordination that didn't provide for them to be filled and emptied by movements of the entire rib cage, instead of only the diaphragm? Given the information presented here, there are no reasons other than ignorance or indifference, as I see it.

Of course (and you're right for thinking so), in real life the matter isn't nearly that calamitous. We do get the O_2 and get rid of the CO_2 in spite of what we know or don't about it. As I say to my students, there are two kinds of breaths in this world, the unconscious ones and the conscious ones, and the former far outnumber the latter. Nature has ensured that this process go on more-or-less automatically for as long as life continues. But this is really not an excuse for not giving due attention to how this vital (Latin—*vīta*, life) process takes place and how we might enhance it.

How the process takes place has been the subject, as best I could manage it, of all of the foregoing; suggesting that it might be enhanced provokes a demand (or at least a polite request), to know "Why?" Here are some of the major physiological reasons:

1. All circulatory and blood-quality aspects of bodily function are enhanced as more lung tissue is utilized.
2. There is more space in the rib cage and therefore less pressure on the contents, namely lungs and heart.
3. The heart is generally supported higher in the body, lessening the distance between it and the brain, and thus reducing pumping effort.
4. The opening and closing of the rib cage—think of a bellows—in itself functions as a large pump complementing the pumping action of the heart.

Something I want to make very clear here is that nothing advocated in this chapter is a "breathing exercise." If that is what you seek, you may find many, many such in books, websites, and classes on yoga, t'ai chi, chi kung, and other systems. Exercise in the sense of special activities for special purposes is not my thing. What *is* my thing is normal posturality, and what I have tried to show is how such a normal (Lengthened) posturality includes enhancement of the respiratory function, as well as every other metabolic function. Take it as a maxim, like any structure, *we function best at our full structural dimension.*

I would be remiss not to re-emphasize that most of our breaths are unconscious and reflex ones—the only ones that we can modify are those of which we become aware. And the only ones of which we become aware result from the curious phenomenon of *remembering*. Strangely enough, remembering is something that we ultimately cannot force ourselves to do, in spite of all the strings-around-fingers and latest technological gadgets that go off at regular or random intervals. True remembering is a function of *wanting*—Freud said it so well in observing that the lover does not forget his appointment! So if we are interested in the benefits—or more modestly, some of the experiences—of a normal posturality, we have to *remember* actually to use ourselves in new and non-habitual ways according to principles that we only provisionally accept until validated by our experience. Only through the risky investment of practice can come skill.

Also I say again that this book is not intended for self-instruction in any comprehensive sense—there are simply too many individual variables, both in constitution and acquired habit, to provide the necessary detail. Anyone who has ever felt the need for and actually had lessons from a good teacher in any skill whatever will understand this. That said, I will close the chapter by describing a means of beginning to explore the concepts I've here advanced.

Lie on your back on the floor with your knees drawn up comfortably, soles of feet on floor, and enough support under your head (books, firm pillow) to keep it more-or-less level relative to your torso. Place your hands on your lower rib cage, elbows out to the side, and notice what you feel as you breathe "normally" (that is, without any attempt to change). Now try not to move your rib cage at all as you take in a gently filling breath—this is not an athletic event—a slight pressure inward of your hands may help at first. When you're successful at this coordination, you will perceive a pronounced upward movement of your entire abdominal area, and you will be experiencing the "breathe from your diaphragm" mode of respiration. Do it a few times to clarify both the movement and the experience. Now, leaving one hand on your lower rib cage, put the other on your lower abdomen between navel and pubis, and form the intention of taking a breath in without letting the lower abdomen rise at all. When you realize (make real) this intention (it may take awhile), you will perceive a pronounced outward and upward movement of your rib cage, and you will be experiencing the "breath as postural process" mode, with the exception that, due to gravity in the supine position, the release and outward movement of the upper abdominal musculature will likely be hardly perceptible or not at all. Naturally, practice tends to improve performance, so do both modes alternately a few times while still lying down.

Come back to standing, placing one hand over the area between your navel and rib cage and the other between your navel and pubis. "Suck in your gut" a few times, tightening the muscles under both hands, and noticing how you move and how it feels. Now let that go, and try just pulling your lower abdominals inward an inch or so, and holding them there while breathing in (again, this may take one, a few, or many trials). When you are successful at maintaining the inward focus of your lower abdominals on a gently filling inbreath, then try allowing the area under your upper hand simultaneously to release and move forward. At first it may well feel like "you can't get there from here," or like rubbing your head and patting your stomach at the same time, but I promise the coordination is there for you. When you're successful, you will be experiencing the first bloom of a practice that can lead you, in my experience, to a new level of psycho-physical well-being.

Just to be clear, it's not a question of breathing either one way or the other of the two modes discussed here as we go through our days—that would be perfectionistic and unproductive, in addition to impossible. It's rather a matter of developing awareness in an important skill and being able to perform it when we remember it because we choose to do so. You might reasonably ask, "Well, gee, how many of these Optimal Metabolic Breaths would I need in a day to do me any good?" and my answer to you would have to be, "Honestly, I don't know." For myself, however, my answer is that every single one taken is one more than would have otherwise been the case—a step in the right direction. Such is the nature of process, in postural action as well as in financial investing and all the other things we do in the hope of return—faith by whatever name is never far from us in the pursuit of happiness, including health and well-being.

8 Where Do We Go from Here?

At this point, after quite a bit of conceptual buffeting, you hopefully have a fuller understanding than previously of a normal posturality, both of what it is and why it matters. Perhaps you've even had intimations of such a posturality in yourself through the experiential explorations that I've suggested. Now you've arrived where, in a yellow woods of your being, two paths diverge. The one taken (or *not*, as Frost so poignantly put it) can make, if not *all* the difference, at least a considerable difference in your life. Essentially, the one path you follow by yourself and the other in the company of a guide, at least for a time.[1] Regardless of which, however, some notion of what you may encounter on the way may be helpful, and to that end I devote this chapter to a look at some major therapeutic and educational approaches to problems of musculoskeletal provenance—mainly pain, tension, and fatigue—for which postural change is deemed desirable. To start, please re-read §§3–5, and particularly §5, for it is in the understanding of posture as a *constant, unified, and psycho-physical process* that any approach to postural improvement must be assessed.

---

[1] Not that this particular choice (unlike some) is irrevocable—as the *brujo* (medicine man, sorcerer) Don Juan said, you may always leave and return to a "path with heart" (Carlos Castaneda, *The Teachings of Don Juan: A Yaqui Way of Knowledge*, Ballantine Books, 1968).

Three distinct approaches in this field may be termed 1) Manipulation, 2) Exercise, and 3) Awareness. Although these approaches in modern practice are by no means mutually exclusive, the classical forms of their exemplars to be discussed show clearly the distinctions I wish to make. Thus, I will be remarking on some major current representatives of each approach, but it should be understood that each has many "schools" and variations, very much like religious sects in their proliferation and particularization. In any case, my concern is with principles more than individual programs; hopefully you will find these principles useful in your thinking on these matters. Thus, under Manipulation we'll look at chiropractic, massage therapy, and rolfing.[2] Exercise will include physical therapy, yoga, and Pilates. Awareness is represented by the Alexander Technique, the Feldenkrais Method, and muscle biofeedback.

Manipulation

Chiropractic—The working theory of the traditional chiropractor is that pressure on nerves, especially spinal nerves, is responsible for many of the ills of humankind. This pressure is caused by the misalignment of spinal vertebrae, called "subluxations," and is treated by more-or-less forceful manipulation of the spine, which, through

---

[2] Ida P. Rolf, Ph.D., was explicit without explanation, at least in titling her book, that "rolfing" be spelled in lower case (See Note 4, p. 66).

restoring normal alignment, putatively relieves nerve pressure and restores normal function. Typically, initial adjustments don't "hold," requiring the patient to return for many more in the hope of cure. Indeed, chiropractors freely expound the importance of regular adjustments on a permanent basis for prevention as well as amelioration of symptoms. Historically, posture has been a secondary concern for them, and if improvement is noted, it is considered a natural result of treating the all-important subluxation.[3]

Massage Therapy—The central principle of all types of massage therapy is that the symptoms for which the client is seeking relief result from various imbalances in soft tissue itself, chiefly muscle in traditional Western systems but also organs, and that manipulation of various types—rubbing, kneading, patting, etc.—applied directly to both the tissue in question and the body in general brings relief by structural loosening and increase of circulation. As with chiropractic, beneficial postural change is viewed as a by-product of the treatment process rather than being explicitly sought or advocated.

---

[3] See, for example, David Seaman and Steve Troyanovich, "The Chasm Between Posture and Chiropractic Education and Treatment," *Dynamic Chiropractic* (Vol. 18, Issue 01). Retrieved from (http://www.dynamicchiropractic.com/mpacms/dc/article.php?id=31485).

Rolfing—One of the leading "name-brands" of the modern scene, it was the creation of Ida Rolf, Ph.D. (1896–1979), whose original training was in biochemistry and physiology. Her book is a lucid and thorough description of the human situation from the viewpoint of both bodily structure in general and in the light of her approach to structural problems.[4] Rolf believed that postural misalignments and distortions were the result of the skeletal musculature's being held to incorrect positions and movements by overly contracted *fascia*, the fibrous tissues between the muscles and forming the sheaths of muscles. Her therapy to undo these contractures and restore normal function consisted of deep, sometimes very deep, manipulation of the musculature, sometimes using techniques, such as a forcefully applied elbow, considerably removed from those of traditional massage.[5] In any case, rolfing, unlike chiropractic or massage therapy, seeks postural improvement—"structural integration"—as a direct result rather than as a by-product of the treatment process.

The essence of manipulative approaches is that clients **receive** *a treatment which is supposed to* **relieve** *their problem.*

---

[4] Ida P. Rolf, *rolfing: The Integration of Human Structures* (New York: Harper & Row, 1977).
[5] In discussing clients' experience of this process, Rolf was perhaps showing a wry sense of humor (or perhaps *not*) in titling one of her chapters "Many People Refer to This Drama as Pain"!

Exercise

Physical Therapy—The premise of physical therapy is that imbalances in muscle action—some too weak, some too strong, some too short, some too long—lead to the problems for which the therapy is prescribed. Typically after referral by a physician, the therapist performs a qualitative analysis[6] of the patient's condition, using both the physician's diagnosis and various techniques such as muscle testing, and based on that analysis, prescribes exercises—structured movements—to ameliorate symptoms and restore normal function. The salient factors in this process, which in practice vary widely, are the accuracy of the therapist's analysis, the appropriateness of the prescribed exercises, and the quality of the patient's performance of them.

Yoga—Hatha yoga (one of several major traditions of this discipline) is widely understood and practiced as a system of psycho-physical culture having for its purpose the improvement and maintenance of health through the systematic performance of various postures or *asanas*. These postures of ancient origin are thought to have and, in the experience of many, do have beneficial psycho-physical effects—relaxation, pain relief, focus, calmness, etc. In spite of its psychological dimension, I characterize

---

[6] Qualitative analysis refers to inferences about muscular action based on physiological knowledge, observation of the patient, and implicational—"if-then"—reasoning.

yoga as an Exercise approach because its method requires the repetition of arbitrary movements[7]—postures—for desired results. For the client or student, a choice must be made, regardless of therapeutic aim, among the manifold postures of the yogic armamentarium. And, like physical therapy, the quality of this choice—how well or not it actually addresses the conditions at hand—depends on the knowledge, experience, and (let us not forget) talent of the person—yoga teacher or other—making it. Here it must be said that while many and perhaps most of these postures are benign or at least neutral in their effects on the body, some are positively harmful and should be avoided because of their deleterious effects on the spine. These harmful postures especially include all that involve cervical and/or lumbar flexion (reversing the normal inward curve) combined with weight-bearing, common ones being the plow, the shoulder stand, and the bicycle.[8] Under such conditions, repetitive by the nature of the discipline, the discs are squeezed back toward the nerves emerging from the spinal cord at each vertebra.[9] Regardless of the stimulation of chakras or other possible benefit, the spine does not much like to be bent around a

---

[7] By "arbitrary" I mean prescribed or non-naturalistic, in contrast to what I've called "existential movement," such as standing, walking, sitting, etc. (pp. 34–35).

[8] The classical Western calisthenic of touching the toes with the knees straight is also a notorious member of this club.

[9] Judy Alter's, *Surviving Exercise* (Boston: Houghton-Mifflin, 1983) is a very fine resource for those who want to do exercises without hurting themselves.

lot (pp. 36–40); think about what would happen if you took a wire coat hanger and bent it back and forth repeatedly if these types of postures tempt you.[10]

Pilates—Named after founder Joseph Pilates (1883–1967), originally a gymnast, boxer, and overall physical-culturist, the Pilates Method is currently the most popular of the "name-brand" practices, probably succeeding Feldenkrais (see below) in that regard. Pilates believed that conditions of the modern sedentary lifestyle fomented bad posture, poor breathing, and general physical debility, which he addressed through exercises designed to build up the deep muscles of the torso, the "core." He invented specialized machines—"Reformers"—that typify a Pilates studio to facilitate this enterprise, the concept being to hold some parts of the body immobile in order to develop the deep torso musculature through isolation techniques. Pilates differs from physical therapy in its emphasis on overall physical improvement rather than on specific clinical symptoms, and from yoga in that postural proficiency is a direct goal rather than a by-product. Also differing from yoga is that the Pilates regimen, while offered in many variations, is a relatively homogeneous one, not characterized by a yoga-like array of postures from which a coherent program must be assembled.

---

[10] Recent support for my argument is found in William J. Broad, "How Yoga Can Wreck Your Body" (*New York Times Magazine*, January 8, 2012).

*The essence of exercise approaches is that clients **perform** arbitrary actions that someone else **prescribes**.*

Awareness

The Alexander Technique—Radically different from any of the other approaches here discussed, Alexander employs neither manipulation nor exercise in the pursuit of its aim, which is the restoration of a satisfactory "use of the self," the key conception of F. M. Alexander (1869–1955). He saw the problem as one of faulty patterns of bodily support and movement, acquired unconsciously and perpetuated by habit, the remedy for which was bringing these patterns to conscious awareness in order to inhibit or "not-do" them in the normal activities of daily life. His method, followed by Alexander teachers to this day, consisted of guiding a pupil (or student, not client or patient) to an unfamiliar but correct performance of a totally familiar but habitual act, such as rising from a chair (or standing, sitting, walking, or taking breath). The sensory contrast between familiar and unfamiliar—in alignment, balance, or effort—revealed the underlying habit, and awareness of the actual habit opened the path for its modification through inhibition in real-time action. Although the main teaching of the Alexander Technique—awareness of habit in the pursuit of a normal posturality—is universal in principle, it is elusive in practice, primarily because of the sheer force of decades of accumulated habit and the necessity for students to embrace process rather than results in their efforts, not only initially but ongoingly. Alexander teachers are also relatively scarce, being concentrated for the most part in metropolitan areas.

The Feldenkrais Method—In terms of the present discussion, the work developed by Moshe Feldenkrais is a kind of hybrid, having aspects of both Exercise—in that arbitrary movements are performed—and Awareness—in that hundreds of ingenious movements—far from ordinary calisthenics—are designed to create *Awareness Through Movement.*[11] In its original form the method involved trained instructors giving detailed directions for these movements to classes of floor-lying clients— Feldenkrais being a strong advocate of group rather than individual instruction—who executed the directions to the best of their ability without forcing. Often done on one side of the body only, Feldenkrais' hypothesis was that the passive side "learned" from the performing side. His basic conception was that of "re-programming" the brain's movement centers to a normal posturality through the repetition over time of a sufficient variety of these movements. Later on, to the original Awareness Through Movement classes were added individual lessons in Functional Integration, perhaps in recognition that both subject matter and learners sometimes require the immediacy and detail of the private session, in spite of Feldenkrais' early declaration that "... re-education has

---

[11] Moshe Feldenkrais (New York: Harper & Row, 1972).

much better prospects of success if conducted in groups and not in the seclusion and pretended secrecy of the consulting room."[12]

Muscle Biofeedback—In this approach, which one author characterized as an "electronic Alexander Technique,"[13] technology comes to the aid of the human observer. The technique of Surface Electromyography (sEMG) electronically registers changes in muscular activity at a location of interest by means of sensors attached to the skin over the muscle, and outputs these changes as visible or audible signals, the "feedback." After establishing a baseline level, increased and often excessive levels of muscular activity are thus communicated to the subject. It is often the case that the subject will not have been previously aware of what and how much muscle action has been employed in a given task that may have produced discomfort, such as "mousing" at the computer. By monitoring the output signals in real time, subjects can sometimes reduce these excessive efforts through a process of consciously attending to the signals with the intention that they slow down or otherwise diminish. The teacher-therapist may also facilitate postural changes that result in reduced efforts. A great advantage of sEMG in the field of postural education and therapy is that subjects/clients/patients get objective

---

[12] *Body and Mature Behavior* (New York: International Universities Press, 1949), p. 163.
[13] Michael Gelb, *Body Learning* (New York: Henry Holt, 1987), p. 146.

information in real time—awareness—about how they are managing specific tasks. It is not clear how such information would be gathered or used for the purpose of improving overall posturality; obviously a great deal—as in all approaches, truth be told—depends on the individual teacher-therapist.[14]

The essence of awareness approaches is that, in order to **change** *habitual behavior, one must* **know** *in real time what that behavior actually is.*[15]

It is the matter of *habit* that now needs fuller discussion, because it is the least understood as well as the most important aspect of postural education and therapy. Many decades ago, the great American philosopher John Dewey put it this way (the sheer force of the writing demanding full quotation):

A man who does not stand properly forms a habit of standing improperly, a positive, forceful habit. The common implication that his mistake is merely negative, that he is simply failing to do the right thing, and that the failure can be made good by an order of will is absurd. One might as well suppose that the man who is a slave of whiskey-

---

[14] The work of Whatmore and Kohli (Note 2, p. 18) was an early application of this technique. A comprehensive recent source is Erik Peper and Katherine Hughes Gibney, *Muscle Feedback at the Computer* (Warren, MI: Bio-Medical Instruments Inc., 2006).
[15] F. M. Alexander once remarked to a pupil, "The things that don't exist are the most difficult to get rid of."

drinking is merely one who fails to drink water. Conditions have been formed for producing a bad result, and the bad result will occur as long as these conditions exist. They can no more be dismissed by a direct effort of will than the conditions that create drought can be dispelled by whistling for wind. It is as reasonable to expect a fire to go out when it is ordered to stop burning as to suppose that a man can stand straight in consequence of a direct action of thought and desire. The fire can be put out only by changing objective conditions; *it is the same with rectification of bad posture* [my italics].[16]

The "objective conditions" of one's posturality are both physical and psychical in nature; on the physical side is the "hardware"—muscles, nerves, brain, etc.—while on the psychical side is the "software"—information from the central nervous system in the form of neural impulses reflecting both reflex and voluntary activity. In between these two is what might be called, to extend the computer analogy, the "firmware," coordinative patterns or "motor programs," which, understood at the necessary level of complexity, may be easily enough viewed as "habits."[17]

---

[16] *Human Nature and Conduct* (New York: Modern Library, 1930), p. 29.
[17] "Firmware" in the computer lexicon refers to programmable hardware; "motor program" is a concept from movement science referring to neural structures that, once acquired through practice, essentially "run" without feedback. Musical scales as executed by an expert performer would be one example of an infinitude of such programs. See J. A. Scott Kelso, Ed., *Human Motor Behavior* (Hillsdale, NJ: Lawrence Erlbaum Associates, 1982), *passim*, esp. Chapters 7 and 8.

Some habits are consciously acquired. One can easily enough recall, for example, or at least reconstruct in one's mind, taking the first cigarette, and then the next, and the next, etc. until the habit is formed. Other habits come unconsciously. Regardless of effort to recall, one cannot remember taking the first step, or saying the first word, or doing the first anything in the domain of existential movement—yet surely the stereotypical behavior has become present and available. It is difficult but necessary to realize that in large part one's very selfhood—and most certainly one's posturality—is manifested only *through*, and by no means simply *in spite of*, these unconscious habits. Strangely enough, the essence of what both Dewey and I are trying to say is perfectly suggested by the old nursery rhyme, "There was a crooked man, and he walked a crooked mile" (or, for present purposes, a *shortened* man who walked a *shortened* mile)!

Postural actions in their ongoing consummations can be only as correct or normal as the underlying habit that ultimately carries them out.

Relative to the three approaches to postural rectification (Manipulation, Exercise, Awareness) discussed here, I hope it would now be clear that while any approach or method may be helpful or effective in terms of relieving symptoms, to the extent that it is exclusively or largely based in addressing less than jointly and fully the hardware, the software, and the firmware, it is incomplete in terms of the larger issue of the posturality of the person. Also needing to be borne in mind is that in the real world of postural practitioners, it is the *individual* teacher or therapist who will have a philosophy and a program inviting assessment according to the criteria developed in this book. I wish you well, Gentle Reader—from what you've read here, from your own research and experience, and, in the spirit of the *brujo* Don Juan[18]—in finding your own "path with heart."

---

[18] Note 1, p. 61.

9 Bibliographic Essay

Having already cited my specific sources in the footnotes, I want in this Bibliographic Essay to treat in a more leisurely fashion some additional works that have been crucial to my thinking and practice over the years—as in Francis Bacon's famous observation, "Some books are to be tasted, some swallowed, and some few to be chewed and digested." I could possibly observe some kind of logical order, but, on balance, think that the job will be better done rather more impressionistically.

I disclosed in my Introduction that I am and have been for a long time a Teacher of the Alexander Technique, thus obviously having a bias, no small part of which was developed by reading. I didn't read Alexander first but rather Wilfred Barlow's *The Alexander Technique* (New York: Knopf, 1973). Barlow was a rheumatologist, and his medically oriented account of the Technique gave conceptual validation to the experiences I was having in lessons. Alexander's writing I first encountered in an anthology put together by Edward Maisel, the only thing readily available at the time (1972), which in its first incarnation was titled (!) *The Resurrection of the Body* (New York: Delta Books, 1969) and often found on the religious or metaphysical shelves in bookstores. Later and understandably re-titled *The Alexander Technique: The Essential Writings of F. Matthias Alexander* (New York: Lyle Stuart,

1990), it featured a 38-page critical introduction by Maisel putting the Technique in an historical and cultural perspective that really has not been surpassed. Of Alexander's four books, the most popular is *The Use of the Self* (New York: Dutton, 1932), but I find his earlier *Constructive Conscious Control of the Individual* (New York: Dutton, 1923) the clearest picture of the method, if not the man. Among the many books now available about the Technique, the one I most often recommend to students is still the late Deborah Caplan's *Back Trouble: A New Approach to Prevention and Recovery* (Gainesville, FL: Triad Publ. Co., 1987), which by virtue of content as opposed to commerce could more accurately have been called "The Alexander Technique: A New Approach to Back Trouble."

A truly pivotal work on my path was Mabel Elsworth Todd's *The Thinking Body: A Study of the Balancing Forces of Dynamic Man* (New York: Paul B. Hoeber, 1937), currently available in reprint. I entered my Alexander certification program as a trainee being schooled in a method; I exited from Todd's book, which I read during training, as a student more of body mechanics than of the often-formulaic procedures of the Alexander Technique per se. In her book, Todd manages a superb narrative account of structures and processes as they operate in space and time, a performance that has inspired my own writing.

Relative to my practice of not only looking at but actually seeing my students (Introduction, p. 1), a book I plucked off a sale table in New York many years ago is *The Body*

Has Its Reasons: Anti-Exercise and Self Awareness.[1] This book, from which I often quote to my students, is an exposition of the teachings of Françoise Mézières, French founder of a method strikingly similar in philosophy to the Alexander Technique though differing in approach. The particular passage I often read aloud is this:

> Classical medical gymnastics is satisfied to analyze and classify the different types of morphology [the branch of biology dealing with structure and form], which are considered constitutional and therefore irreversible. ... Our imperfect structure is considered normal because it's common. ... Françoise Mézières teaches that morphology shouldn't be the science of the classification of dysmorphisms [abnormalities], but *the art of recognizing the perfect form* [my italics], which is the only normal morphology.

The "perfect form" for Mézières, based on her study of ancient Greek sculpture, is what I, perhaps from my raising in rural Iowa, call the "breed standard" (Introduction, Note 1). I tell my students that my job is to see through to their underlying potential through the layers of their habituated development. Thus my work with them can never be a set of fixed procedures or techniques, but can only progress as a path—sometimes clear, sometimes obscure—toward a destination already glimpsed.

---

[1] Thérèse Bertherat and Carol Bernstein (New York: Pantheon Books, 1977).

In subject matter but not essential relevance, I jump to Michael Polanyi's *Personal Knowledge: Towards a Post-Critical Philosophy* (Univ. of Chicago Press, 1962). To me, this is one of those books that everyone who wants to think well should read, not only for the subject matter but also for the sheer exercise of the understanding that it entails. It is 400+ pages of small print organized in numbered sections, and the only way I made it through was to read a section or two a day for several weeks on end. Polanyi took on the task of bridging the supposed gap between science on the one hand and art on the other. He does this brilliantly by demonstrating that "... the act of knowing includes an appraisal; and this personal coefficient, which shapes all factual knowledge, bridges in doing so the disjunction between subjectivity and objectivity."[2] Here I find validation for saying in my Introduction, "Almost always I see at once, because I know how to look."

Speaking of better thinking, I turn, as promised (p. 27), to the *general semantics* of Alfred Korzybski, contained in *Science and Sanity: An Introduction to Non-Aristotelian Systems and General Semantics*, Fifth Edition (Brooklyn, NY: The International Non-Aristotelian Publishing Company, 1950). Korzybski's premise is that certain unconscious habits of inner representation (both to others and self) distort reality and make us "un-sane."

---

[2] P. 17.

Fortunately, one need not invest in the "whole enchilada" of *Science and Sanity* currently at $88.00 (plus shipping) because an excellent presentation is made by Susan Presby Kodish and Bruce I. Kodish in their *Drive Yourself Sane: Using the Uncommon Sense of General Semantics*, Third Edition (Pasadena, CA: Extensional Publishing, 2011).

Getting back to more explicit physicality, I call attention to a work already cited by footnote (Chapter 4, n. 2) but needing fuller discussion, *Essentials of Body Mechanics in Health and Disease*, by four twentieth-century orthopedists highly affiliated in Bostonian (Massachusetts General Hospital, Harvard Medical School) and national medical establishments, namely Joel E. Goldthwait,[3] Lloyd T. Brown, Loring T. Swaim, and John G. Kuhns. Here was their purpose, as given in the Preface to the first edition of 1934:

> With the increasing number of persons afflicted with the chronic diseases, the problem of treatment is becoming more and more difficult for the medical profession, and the results of the diseases causing such conditions are presenting an ever-increasing economic problem both to the patient and to the community.

Sound familiar? They continue:

---

[3] Who, for example, was chief of the U.S. Army Medical Service in World War I.

A steadily increasing segment of older individuals in our population presents to the medical profession a great challenge to maintain the physical fitness and the usefulness of these persons who are more advanced in years. ... For the understanding and relief of these conditions, it is hoped that this publication may suggest new lines of study and treatment, which will prove as helpful to the general practitioner as they have to the authors.

Their "new lines of study and treatment" consisted of the understanding and systematic improvement of the mechanics of the body, and the "proper training of the body so that the best possible state of health may be obtained." Their book consists of analysis of all major systems of the body and how these systems are negatively affected by, to use my language, a subnormal or abnormal posturality. Although their approach to the problem is by my standards crude—conventional posture exercises—their essential grasp and clinical insights would be valuable to anyone pursuing—particularly as a provider—postural education or therapy. Virtually disappeared into the maw of time and fashion, but with undiminished relevance, this book may still be found on that bibliophilic miracle, the Internet.

Because "The Optimal Metabolic Breath" (Chapter 7) is likely the most difficult and also the most controversial aspect of my book, I want to make its sources clear. Let me say right off that I was not taught this coordination by

82

anyone; I arrived at it independently, first through inferences from studies in the works to be cited and then experientially in my own body. Later I found a striking correspondence between it and Alexander's description of breathing coordination,[4] as well as the "reverse" or "prebirth" breath of *t'ai-chi chi-kung* (more on that anon).

It was in Goldthwait et al. (previous paragraph) that I first became aware of the "two abdomens," upper and lower: "It should be noted that these muscles [the abdominals] have two separate nerve supplies. The muscles below the umbilicus can be contracted independently of those above it."[5] To this basic insight were added findings from two studies by a noted authority on respiratory muscle action, A. De Troyer: "Mechanical Action of the Abdominal Muscles" and "Actions of the Respiratory Muscles or How the Chest Wall Moves in Upright Man."[6] These articles allowed me to understand how the diaphragm paradoxically *lifts* the rib cage by *contraction* over the fulcrum of the viscera as stabilized by the lower abdominals.

---

[4] In F. Matthias Alexander, *Man's Supreme Inheritance* (New York: Dutton, 1918, 3rd Printing 1919), Part III, "The Theory and Practice of a New Method of Respiratory Re-education," pp. 331ff.
[5] p. 271.
[6] Both published in the *Bulletin Européen Physiopathologie Respiratoire* (1983, *19*, pp. 575–581) and (1984, *20*, pp. 409–13), resp.

Finally, the series of relevant illustrations in I. A. Kapandji's *The Physiology of the Joints*[7] provided the means for visualizing these complex muscular actions as they take place in real time. Of Kapandji's three-volume work, truly indispensable for the student of posturality, I can do no better than to quote my late colleague Troup Mathews, who characterized it as "... an anatomy text which is notable for its expressively aesthetic illustrations of movement on the one hand, and the clear engineering interpretations of human joint structure and muscular vectors on the other."[8]

The connection to *t'ai-chi chi-kung* mentioned above is from Jou, Tsung Hwa's *The Tao of Tai-Chi Chuan*,[9] where the author says "In Tai-Chi Chuan prebirth breathing is designed to provide the special kind of energy required for rejuvenation. ... Only when the prebirth breathing becomes the normal breathing pattern can the aging process actually be reversed." Be that as it may, I am in full accord that the cultivation of better breathing is a decided health benefit.

Lastly, I wish to bring forward two works which, although separated in time by more than sixty years, are intimately connected both by the yawning chasm between recogni-

---

[7] Second Ed., Vol. Three, *The Trunk and Vertebral Column* (Edinburgh: Churchill Livingstone, 1974), pp. 136–151.
[8] "Parliamentary Procedure & the Breath—Ron Dennis at the AGM," *NASTAT NEWS* (Issue 16, Summer 1992), p. 13.
[9] Warwick, NY: Tai Chi Foundation, 1980, p. 126.

tion and neglect on the one hand, and, on the other, by subject matter and relevance for my own work.

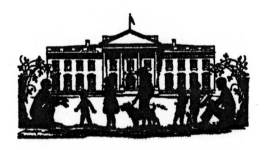

This graphic is from the title page of an obscure work that I photocopied in the Teachers College-Columbia University library, after tracking it down from an equally obscure source. The full title is *Body Mechanics: Education and Practice. Report of the Subcommittee on Orthopedics and Body Mechanics. Robert B. Osgood, M.D., Chairman. White House Conference on Child Health and Protection.* Published in 1932, during the still-waxing Great Depression, and dedicated to "The Children of America, Whose Faces Are Turned Toward the Light of a New Day and Who Must Be Prepared to Meet a Great Adventure," this document faded quickly into the limbo inexorably awaiting most of what is written (and certainly most government reports), but it speaks as clearly today, to those with ears to hear, as when it first came out. Whoever could imagine today a White House Conference on body mechanics?!

The gist of its 166 pages was that, on the basis of considerable empirical data, upwards of 75% of the country's youth exhibited subnormal and potentially symptom-producing grades of body mechanics. Is it likely the figure would be less in today's even more sedentary and tech-nologized society? The Subcommittee, consisting of four male physicians and a female physical hygiene professor, called for widespread instruction in body mechanics ("posture" to you, bub) at virtually every level of public and private education, from kindergartens to medical schools—truly health and not illness care! No isolated phenomenon, the report is a fair example of a body of medical literature from the first half of last century deal-ing with the relationship of body mechanics to health and disease, as exemplified by the work by Goldthwait et al. cited above. The fact that organized medicine has not taken such issues very seriously is not a reliable gauge of their importance, as fashions change in the medical arena as in others. Developments in pharmacology and technol-ogy spurred by World War II, for example, have effectively overshadowed less spectacular but no less basic behav-ioral issues in the field of human well-being.

This work's companion piece in my consciousness is Michele Arsenault's *Moving to Learn: A Classroom Guide to Understanding and Using Good Body Mechanics.* Self-published in 1998, this book, which is a detailed teach-er's manual as well as a personal chronicle, gives the author's experience in teaching elementary school chil-dren from the perspective of both the Alexander Tech-nique and classical science. Through a grant from the Institute for Schools of the Future, Arsenault met weekly with kindergarteners, fourth graders, and fifth graders at a public school on New York City's Lower East Side. As she later wrote, "They are easily engaged and challenged by a subject that has such personal relevance in their lives." Quoting her further: "... five-year olds already exhibit mis-use and a significant decrease in flexibility in their hip and ankle joints ... nine-year olds complain of backaches and neck problems and move and collapse much like their adult counterparts; children have the same misconceptions about their bodies as their teachers." Although Arsenault's work as preserved in *Moving to Learn* has not yet seen—nor, it must be said, is it for the foreseeable future likely to see—the recognition and application it deserves, it stands nevertheless as a shining monument to her dedication as well as, hopefully, a flickering beacon to future travelers, in this neglected but crucial field.

So often in my work with adults, who must in one way or another acquire some semblance of a normal posturality in order to relieve their rebelling bodies, I am told, "If only I could have learned this as a child in school!" Clearly, the full humanitarian potential of postural education, in its moral as well as physical and intellectual aspects, will be realized only when its principles and associated skills are imparted early to the young. Conventional curricula in physical education at any grade level do not remotely address this problem. It seems hopelessly utopian, in this era of economic dislocation, man-made and natural disaster, climate change, and all the rest, to envision a system of early education where children learn along with the three Rs that truly their backs are basic! But if we must so envision, if only perhaps to ward off despair, this work of Arsenault's illuminates a distinct step in that direction by articulating its content at a level and in a form consonant with the mainstream of primary schooling in this country. Would that it were so!

Appendix I ~ Julie O.

By Julie Orta, MPH, MCHES

[My student Julie Orta works for the Centers for Disease Control and Prevention, Atlanta, Georgia. Her story is unusual but not unique in my 30+ year career: to be sure, most of my students have been grateful for their time with me without the drama of Julie's account. I asked her to write it particularly to illustrate how what I "see" as a postural educator and how I use those observations in my work both profit from a comprehensive view of normal posturality. For Julie and many others, appropriate postural education could render unnecessary their huge expense of trouble, treasure, and trauma.]

I am a 41 year old female who appears healthy—I am thin, have energy, sleep well, have relatively low stress levels, and practice a healthy lifestyle. However, I have had a condition for 27 years that has had an impact on my health and quality of life. The term for my condition is "degenerative disc disease" with desiccated, ruptured herniated discs that cause chronic neck and shoulder pain with acute spasms.

A History of My Pain

It started with pain in the right shoulder (trapezius) at age 14 likely due to the repetitive motion of scooping ice cream and decorating ice cream cakes at a part time job. By age 16 it was too painful to hold a head of lettuce out in front of me. By my early 20s as a teacher I was unable to write on the board above waist level. Always there would be what felt like a tight muscle knot on the top of the right shoulder, and over time the left side started to feel sore as well. When taking walks, my left arm would move but the right arm would remain still to avoid aggravation. My first neck spasm did not occur until age 24. I was walking and all of the sudden, my neck got very sore and locked in place. I reclined the rest of the day, unable to turn my head. The next morning I was able to move again but with difficulty and with a huge knot at the same location as the original right shoulder pain, so my assumption was that the neck pain and shoulder pain were related. From that time until now my neck has "gone out" over 20 times. Each time the experience is a stabbing pain that causes immobilization. Usually the outage runs five-ish days in which I'm horizontal for the first two to three days and gradually upright a bit each day after that. When my neck goes out, my head cannot be centered above the neck. (My head generally is stuck jutted forward—like a chicken locked in the "cluck forward" motion—and off to the left side a little.) Wearing a soft neck brace helps with stabilization, but for the first few days the best treatment is to take the load off by lying down, sometimes with a prop under the right shoulder. Although it is typically the right side of the neck that goes out, several times the left side has gone out, and most recently the top of the neck (base of the head) in the center went out, causing headaches across the back of my head.

When health care practitioners have tried to treat my condition or examined the MRI, they have always asked if I had been in a car accident or had some other traumatic injury to the neck or shoulders. The answer is no, and I have a hard time believing that my two years in the ice cream store could have done this. Treatments over the years have included both eastern and western medicine, such as muscle relaxants, 600 mg Gabapentin (nightly), Percocet, steroids (facet joint injections, trigger point injections, cervical epidurals, a Medrol dose pack), acupuncture, acupressure, physical therapy (which threw my neck out), stretching exercises, chiropractics, neuromuscular massage therapy (still doing massage every three-ish weeks), and mostly avoiding any type of activity that would aggravate the condition (e.g., high impact anything, tilting my head up or down for an extended period of time, turning the head to the far right or far left). I even quit playing racquetball, which was the sport I loved and had kept me in great cardiovascular shape for years, because my neck could no longer handle the impact.

In the mid 2000s, facet joint injections provided relief, buying me from a year to a year and a half without a debilitating spasm. By the late 2000s, I graduated to cervical epidurals. In 2011 I had two cervical epidurals, yet within three months of the second epidural, my neck went out again. To date, I have not been a good candidate for surgery primarily because I do not have obvious signs of nerve damage. When my neck generally hurts but isn't in a full blown outage, I take Ibuprofen, but when my neck is out, 800 mg of Ibuprofen provides no relief. When I'm in sheer agony, even Percocet isn't effective. All that is to say, I have been so frustrated from getting only minimal and temporary relief after years of therapies and treatments, having paid thousands of dollars in out-of-pocket expenses and lost productivity.

My Introduction to the Alexander Technique

At the end of 2011 I decided it was time to switch health plans from an HMO to a nationwide PPO that would authorize me to get a full work-up at Mayo Clinic. And that's how I got introduced to the Alexander Technique. My mother used to work with a physician at Mayo Clinic so she connected me with her. I expected her to respond to my condition with the same pessimism as all the other doctors I had encountered over the years. I was wrong. The first thing she did was empathize. The next thing she did was provide a very strong recommendation to get Alexander Technique training, and only afterward if I weren't getting relief, then to arrange for evaluation at Mayo Clinic's multidisciplinary Spine Center. She also suggested, "I think that if you engage in Alexander training, you may not need the Mayo evaluation." Mayo Clinic even has an Alexander Technique instructor on staff.

I confess if the recommendation had come from anyone outside Mayo Clinic, I would have been skeptical about the Alexander Technique because I had never heard of it before, my MRI shows my neck is a mess, and nothing else has worked. But with such a strong conviction coming from a Mayo physician, I was sold. I was directed to a website *www.amsatonline.org/* that provides information about the technique along with a list of certified instructors, and so I contacted the author of this book, Dr. Ron Dennis, and took 10 weekly lessons from him from December 2011 to February 2012. And has my life ever changed!

Improving My Posture

All 10 lessons were valuable, awareness raising, and empowering. But I think I got the most bang for the buck on the first visit, when in the midst of talking to each other, he interrupted and said something to the effect of, "you know, you seem to tense up your shoulders quite a bit." I initially thought to myself, huh? Why would I go out of my way to flex what already hurts all the time. But he was right. My shoulders were tightened up and I had to "force" them to relax. They went down. But then within a moment, they were right back up there again, and I don't remember how that happened. Being tight had become so automatic to me over the years that over the weeks ahead

I would catch myself already in the tightened mode and would have to deliberately relax them.

Every lesson involved learning how to carry my body in ways that would improve my posture. (After all these years, the cure was better posture?) I learned not only how to sit and how to be in the standing position, but also especially how to transition from sitting to standing and vice versa. I had never paid any attention before meeting Ron as to which parts of the body move and how to change that action so that I don't strain my neck or shoulders, but he spent countless attempts showing me how to do it optimally.

One day when I thought I had finally become proactive (instead of reactive) in keeping the shoulders relaxed, I was at my desk at work and realized that every time I tried to write something down on a piece of paper, my shoulder would tighten up again. I wasn't catching myself after the fact; this time I was ahead of the game, fully aware of what was happening. But I was so frustrated because I had no clue how to write without engaging that muscle. So I took it to Ron at my next lesson and he opened up a table, put a piece of paper and pencil in front of me, observed this very regular activity of mine, and coached me to another way of holding the pencil—my shoulder tension was starting in my hand and fingers! Now I'm also able to drive and turn the steering wheel without aggravating the shoulder, something I couldn't do before my Alexander lessons.

Sometimes I feel like I have reverted back to early childhood, learning how to write, sit, stand, and bend (fold, as he calls it), and in a sense I have. I'm finally undoing bad habits that formed more than 30 years ago. He spent a lot of time teaching me about lengthening as well. And I've known for years I should do what I thought was "suck in my gut," but Ron gave me a new coordination for that action and a new, far more important reason for it that goes way beyond aesthetics...even how we breathe is part of improved posture. *[Julie speaks here of the Optimal Metabolic Breath, discussed in Chapter 7.]*

One day I said all animated to Ron at the beginning of the lesson, "I can't believe how much posture matters in pain management!" I mean really, after all these years all I needed to do was hold my body better? Is it too good to be true? Well, I think I have the answer. One day I was working from home and decided to work seated on the sofa with my laptop on my lap instead of seated at the desk using a desktop computer. For the several hours that I sat on the couch, I knew I had bad posture, but I didn't bother to correct it because it was just easier to stay where I was. My left arm was propped up on the arm rest, my head was tilted down to see the laptop, and my back was twisted slightly because of the left arm on the arm rest. I could tell within the first hour that my neck was starting to hurt but I paid no attention because really, how much could a couple hours of "being naughty" really hurt? The answer is, it hurt for two days straight.

My neck was back to its old self, tight, hard to turn, on the verge of another spasm. I learned my lesson. Posture really does matter.

A New Person

Only time will tell if the Alexander Technique is all I needed and if I'll be spasm-free for as long as I keep practicing the Technique. Even now I'm not 100% pain-free, but I'm pretty close, far closer than I have been in many years. I even played racquetball once and my neck handled it fine. (My heart was another story after three years of pain-induced physical inactivity!) Even if I do have more spasms in the future, I'm confident that continuing to practice the Alexander Technique will decrease their frequency. And in between spasms I'm like a new person, set free from the nagging, around-the-clock pain—let alone the fear of being on the brink of another full blown outage.

Now if only the insurance plans out in the world would embrace and endorse this simple but logical approach to wellness and pain management, they would save tons of money and their patients could get on with their lives a lot faster and with a lot more success.

Update: As of February 2013, one year after finishing my lessons with Ron, I'm proud to say I'm still feeling well. I'm doing strength training and light jogging, and most of all am enjoying life to the fullest!

Appendix II ~ Poise and the Art of Lengthening

In his Foreword to this book, John Austin referred to "poise" as an attribute of normal posturality, prompting me to re-visit this article I wrote more than 20 years ago. "Poise" in this sense may be considered as normal posturality with an additional connotation of readiness, or on-the-vergeness—a kind of labile response-ability—in the crucial moment where an habitual response may be inhibited ("pause and organize") or not. The title derives mainly from Eugen Herrigel's Zen and the Art of Archery,* *a slim volume of 90 pages that in the 1960s and 70s enjoyed wide currency among readers of a certain stripe, among them Alexander folk, dealing eloquently as it did with the practice in traditional Japanese archery of attending mindfully (Note 4, below) to process while pursuing the ostensible goal of hitting a target. In keeping steadfastly to this process, as Herrigel (1884–1955) put it, "fundamentally the marksman aims at himself." I decided to include this piece of mine as an appendix not only because it rings the changes on the main themes of my book, but also because, in the last paragraph, it opens the prospect of Lengthening not only as psycho-physical but also as spiritual enterprise.*

*And also from Raymond Dart's "The Attainment of Poise," see Note 1, below.

"Poise" is a curious word. A bit regal in tone and suggesting nowadays a certain personal command, it originated more prosaically in the language of weights and measures.[1] It can be traced back through the Middle English and Old French *pois*, "weight," to the Latin *pensum*, something weighed, and *pendere*, to weigh. Thus, poise has its etymological basis not primarily in a mental state, but in definite physical action, a specific balancing of mass for mass, as in acrobatics, tight-rope walking, and similar skilled performances.

Perhaps few would consider standing up on two legs a particularly skilled performance, but it is in fact a most prodigious balancing act, as you can verify through recalling the infant's concentrated struggle to master it. Yet how many adults have a concern for, or even an intimation of, the distribution of their various body weights—head, arms, trunk, legs—over their base of support and around their center of gravity? For if these weights—the heaviest that most of us are ever required to lift—are not maintained in balance relative to each other within fairly narrow limits, the resulting strain on muscles, ligaments, and joints to keep the body upright leads inexorably toward the creaks, aches, and fatigue that all-too-familiarly herald and accompany the advancing years.

---

[1]R. A. Dart, "The Attainment of Poise," *South African Medical Journal* (21, 1947), pp. 74–91.

From this point of view, we should see poise as an active, whole-person process, an efficient managing of body weights, with an eye to what has been called structural hygiene.[2] The hygiene of poise is clearly what J. E. Goldthwait, M.D., a former president of the American Orthopedic Association, had in mind in saying:

> An individual is in the best health only when the body is so used that there is no strain on any of its parts. This means that, when standing, the body is held fully erect, with no strain on the joints, the bones, the ligaments, the muscles or any other structures. There should be adequate room for all the viscera, so that their function can be performed normally unless there be some congenital defect.[3]

One might thus be led to think that poise is simply a matter of standing up straight and being done with it. Reality will prove otherwise. Resolve for a day to "stand up straight" and generally attend to the use of your body. You will find embarrassingly few moments of awareness during the day's full round, and you will find that whatever change you can bring to bear in one position disappears as you move to another.

The attainment of poise is rather a matter of learning the art of lengthening. Lengthening means pre-eminently that in standing, sitting, walking, bending, or any activity

---

[2] M.E. Todd, *The Thinking Body* (Hoeber, 1937), pp. 41–42.
[3] J. E. Goldthwait et al., *Essentials of Body Mechanics in Health and Disease*, 5th Ed. (Lippincott, 1952), p. 1.

whatever, one must prevent both unnecessary muscular effort and the very common distortions of the natural curves of the spine. Encompassing a broad field of knowledge and practice, lengthening is an art rather than a precise technique because it involves skill and the application of principle on the basis of experience as contrasted with rigid adherence to arbitrary rules or so-called correct positions.[4,5] It should also be added that lengthening is a process practiced primarily by and not on the individual.

Obviously, the giving of precise, or even of general instructions is beyond words alone, so here a hint must suffice. One first experiences lengthening, usually with the aid of a teacher, and then, like a gardener, one cultivates the conditions that tend to promote it. Much as a wind player keeps the breath going or a string player the bow, in lengthening one sustains the muscular tone that keeps the body up while inhibiting that which pulls it down. Indeed, the great secret is not to be pulling or falling *down* on one's *up*, a principle that may be seen by some to extend further than the present discussion.

It is crucial—though at the outset virtually impossible—to realize that one's lifelong habits, in both thought and action, form the sole standard of what feels right and

---

[4] E. Langer, *Mindfulness* (Addison-Wesley, 1990), p. 6.
[5] F. Matthias Alexander, *Constructive Conscious Control of the Individual* (Methuen, 1924), p. 110.

correct within the self.[6] Against this omnipresent background, new responses are bound to seem unfamiliar, sometimes startlingly so. Students of lengthening can thus easily find themselves in the strange situation of being right and feeling wrong, quite the reverse of the usual order of things. It is in confronting this paradox in all its implications, and in the inevitable encounter of desire, habit, and the will that arises in all serious practice, that one has the possibility of gaining not only that which was initially sought but something more, an inner process of knowing at once dependent upon yet transcending the original goal.

---

[6] Alexander, *The Use of the Self* (Dutton, 1932), Chapter 1, "Evolution of a Technique."

Appendix III ~ Muscles and Mentals: Why We Get Tense

As defined in §1 of Conceptual Foundations (p. 7), "Posture comprises the flow through space and time of all activity of bodily support and movement in the course of living." Ultimately, the source of all this activity is muscular action, but not all muscular action efficiently serves bodily support and movement. Generally, the type of muscular action that compromises normal posturality is called "tension," and it is important to realize that there are two sources of tension in our bodies, mechanical and emotional.

Mechanical tension, mostly the subject of this book, partially results from incorrect body mechanics—poor posture, as commonly called. If bodily segments aren't arranged efficiently relative to the center of gravity and base of support, then balance in upright posture must be maintained by compensatory muscular action. Muscles, in these cases, take over some of the load that should be carried by bones, and thus have to work harder than necessary, resulting in what we experience as tension. There is also mechanical tension resulting from *errors of technique,* where the way one has learned to perform the myriad tasks of civilized life is simply wrong, or at least inefficient. Muscles so used become and remain tense.

This is the kind of tension that bedeviled Julie Orta, as detailed in her story in Appendix I.

Emotional tension results from certain responses based largely in fear that cause us to tighten and hold our muscles protectively, against perceived threats or dangers. In the non-human animal kingdom, under natural conditions, emotional tension probably does not exist because fear results in "fight or flight" responses, and the necessary muscular action is discharged functionally in real time. But in humans, the threats of civilized life rarely require or permit such direct action. A performer experiencing stage fright, a spouse suspecting infidelity, or a worker faced with job loss really can neither fight nor flee in their situations, even though their bodies, through the sympathetic nervous system (adrenalin, etc.) are reacting in varying degrees of survival mode, stimulating the musculature among other emergency responses such as raising the blood pressure, inhibiting peristalsis (digestive action), and closing the sphincters. There is thus brought about tension of varying types, degrees, and durations, and, while it is true that Lengthening out of shortened and tense musculature is always called for, it's also my experience that tension of mechanical origin more than that of emotional origin usually responds more readily to the approach of postural education as presented in this book.

Implications of the foregoing are both cautionary and hopeful for both postural educators/therapists and their students/clients. On the cautionary side, it should be mutually recognized that normal posturality has a psychological and emotional dimension as well as a physical and mechanical one. Professionally, the postural educator-therapist will properly be working primarily in terms of the latter, but not without knowledge and sensitivity concerning the former. On the hopeful side, it should also be recognized that the real person, *here present*, is *one*: the mechanical and the emotional cannot be teased apart, as in the dissecting room, and positive change in one direction is potentially salutary in other directions as well.

The point is nicely illustrated in an unlikely source, Richard Henry Dana's salty account of 19th-century seafaring in *Two Years Before the Mast*:

> There is such a connection between different parts of a vessel, that one rope can seldom be touched without altering another. You cannot stay a mast aft by the back stays, without slacking up the head stays, etc., etc.

The two etceteras at the end of the second sentence by no means reflect authorial laziness, but rather point to manifold and dependent interconnections. Like our muscles and mentals.

About the Author

Son of a chiropractor, Ron Dennis (b. 1937) grew up in a small central-Iowa town in the 1940s and 50s. His involvement with music and the clarinet began one sunny autumn afternoon in fourth grade when, on returning from school, he was presented by his dad with a long, skinny black box. Asking "What's that?" he was told, "Ronald, that's your new clarinet," to which he replied, "I don't want any old clarinet." But one thing led to another, eventually to a degree in music education and ultimately to a position of Principal Clarinet with The Saint Paul Chamber Orchestra, a chair he held for seven years (1969–1976).

Encountering the Alexander Technique in 1972 in Minneapolis, he left the orchestra to train as a teacher of this work—was "called," one could say—being certified in 1979 at the American Center for the Alexander Technique in New York City. During the 80s he pioneered group Alexander instruction there, as well as maintaining a private practice and, beginning in 1982, teaching the Technique at The Juilliard School. During this period he also completed his doctorate (1987) at Teachers College-Columbia University, with Dr. John Austin, who contributed this book's Foreword, as his principal dissertation adviser. Becoming the Technique's "man in Atlanta" in 1990, he has since devoted his professional time to private practice and writing, as well as being active in AmSAT, The American Society for the Alexander Technique. His research paper on balance in normal older women (*Journal of Gerontology:MEDICAL SCIENCES*, 1999, Vol. 54A, No. 1, M8–M11), the first controlled study with "Alexander Technique" in the title to enter the *Index Medicus*, placed the Technique in the global world of scientific research.

After a long and checkered relationship, he finally "divorced" the clarinet in 2002 (now2016 "reconciled") and currently spends his musical energies staying in shape on the ol' licorice stick as well strumming on his harpsichord and on flamenco guitars he builds himself. With his wife Dr. Solange Bonnet (d. 2015, *R.I.P.*) he has been since 2001 a devoted tango dancer.

Index

rolfing   64n., 66